Beyond Natural Cures

Beyond Natural Cures

Naturopathic Psychotherapy:

Ridding Our Lives of Chronic Disease

By: Dr. Aurore Henze Adamkiewicz

Edited by: Nicole Hemsoth

Michigan, USA
Beyond Natural Cures
© 2006 by Aurore (Henze)
Adamkiewicz

All rights reserved. ISBN:

978-0-557-09790-6

LCCN: TXu1-319-549

Second Edition 2009

Printed in the United States of America

Disclaimer:

No part of this book is intended to diagnose or discourage medical treatment. If you are sick please visit a medical doctor and follow your prescribed treatment.

No part of this book can be copied or reproduced in any manner without permission from the publisher.

Dr. Aurore is a doctor of natural health and not a licensed psychologist or medical doctor.

This book is dedicated to:

My Children,
You healed *me* with your love.

To My Husband Randy,
My love through the years

My Dear Friend Tara
Who woke me up and gave me Truth.

Psychologist, Dr. Daniel Schiff
Thank you for training me and believing in me

My midwife, mentor and teacher, Aviva Romm,
Thank you for accepting me and changing my life

Author and Scientist, Dr. James De Meo,
Thank you for saving me from myself.

Asst. Professor of Music at UofM Flint, Brian DiBlassio
Thank you for the gift of music and patience

And, everyone who wants to be free….

*"Am I part of the cure,
Or am I part of the disease?"*

-Coldplay

Table of Contents

Introduction xiii

Chapter 1

The Medical Kingdom and its Lowly Subjects 1

Chapter 2

Healing the Body, Healing the Mind 21

Chapter 3

Naturopathy: Where it's Going, Where it's Gone… 47

Chapter 4

Ancient Healing Meets New Disease 65

Chapter 5

The Aurore Healing Method: 99

Chapter 6

Healing Children Simply: With Color, Sound and Sleep 117

Chapter 7

Naturopathic Psychotherapy: the Time has Come 129

References 147

Resources 152

Introduction

Many Americans have read or are at least familiar with the book *Natural Cures* by Kevin Trudeau. Many of us have been busy self-healing and clearing an array of herbs and vitamins off the shelves of our local health food stores. While this is a tremendous step forward for a society that has, until now, refused to be weaned from pharmaceutical drugs, we have entered into a transitional period, an in-between state in our national health crisis. Many of us are earnestly trying to live a more naturopathic life and are not getting the desired results. Some of us are getting positive results symptomatically in a few areas but are still plagued by a chronic disease or sickness. Then there are those who have become sick, tried taking a popular natural remedy like echinacea and ginger, and when it "didn't work," headed back to the web of medical doctors. These people, I would argue, never fully committed themselves to the naturopathic realm and their skepticism and fear led them to experience flawed results.

    On a positive note, our society is finally breaking free of some of its medical constraints, in part because of rising health care costs and the lack of positive results in current medical treatment. When we start to see our hard-earned money flooding directly to doctors who have harmed our children and families, we begin to understand that we must start reclaiming our power—our right to be healthy and free. For a time, the health insurance companies helped to placate people with the belief that their health care was "free" but this is a fallacy because most health care money is taken from the individual before he or she even sees it. Many people have continued going to doctors, knowing they were not getting what they needed, simply because it was covered by insurance.

    I was happy to see that the book *Natural Cures* caught on so quickly. Trudeau is not the first person to write a book of this nature. He was able to hit the market at a pivotal time and dedicated a considerable amount of money for promoting and advertising. My book, however, takes natural health alternatives a step further by addressing the issue of how to remove blocks to healing and of equal importance, how to find the elusive sense of balance. When discussing blocks to healing, I am referring to both a physical constitutional condition which is also referred to as a chronic miasm in addition to the emotional blocks that can be both conscious and unconscious.

Having exhausted their "natural" resources, many have become hooked on an endless array of expensive supplements without realizing that vitamins and herbs can be as addictive as prescription drugs. Why all this wheel spinning in the natural health realm? It seems to me that there are two issues that are directly responsible for this: isolated, vigilante natural health care professionals and endless self-diagnosing.

The first problem lies in the reality that many naturopath doctors tend to be locked into sedentary alternative healing methods. In some ways, they have become like medical doctors, catching on to a certain trend or mindset and treating each person in the same manner. They can do this easily with special machines, outdated protocols and one-size-fits-all diets. For this subset of practitioners, healing thus becomes a "no brainer."

This can also be said about chiropractors who continually overextend the boundaries of their expertise. It is not unusual to leave their office after they have put on a quick applied kinesiology show and spend at least $200 or more on their special herbs and vitamins, affectionately called "nutri-ceuticals." Like a medical doctor, they rely heavily on radiation (x-rays) and many take a condescending approach to their clients, talking down to them. Rarely do they take the time to sit down with you to educate you about any of the treatment—the relationship is simple to them; they have the information and you are required to benefit from it without understanding any of it at all. Keep in mind, by the way, that the word *doctor* comes from the Latin word *docere*, which means to "teach". In this respect, they make up a segment of border-line natural healthers who have left the cadre of traditional medical doctors but are also too intimidated to step fully into the holistic realm.

Introduction

I pose this question about chiropractic care, "Does one ever get healed from chiropractic treatments?" Once you go to a chiropractor, you will have to keep returning to him or her for the rest of your life. This not because chiropractic care does not work, in fact, it does work by moving your vertebrae and realigning your body. However, many times the relief you experience from a chiropractic treatment is short-lived because the fascia and muscle that has memory in it will clamp down around the bones and put them back to where they were before. Truly the best chiropractors are the ones that specialize in their field, do not rely heavily on x-rays, and incorporate muscle release therapy (be it Rolfing, craniosacral therapy, massage, or myofascial release). A good chiropractor, like any professional, will know his or her limits and will be involved in a community of skilled alternative therapists rather than isolated from them.

I have had my own experiences with chiropractors following chronic paralyzing stiff necks for years after my Orgonomy sessions (an alternative form of psychotherapy). Energy was stuck in my neck, literally and my local chiropractor worked on me for two years trying to correct it. At one point he started threatening me. He said that I had a permanent reverse curve and that if I didn't get x-rays that he wouldn't treat me anymore. I finally went to Rolfing to cure it and yes, it did completely cure it by the way.

Ironically, when I initially told my chiropractor I was going to get Rolfed he discouraged me from doing so and warned me that it was too painful to endure. Later, when he asked me why I don't go back to his office any longer and I told him my neck pain was cured from Rolfing, he admitted he had been Rolfed too! As you can imagine, I was shocked to find out he had gone through all ten of the Rolfing sessions himself. It turns out this practice changed his life and healed his chronic pain but he doesn't recommend it to everybody *because people can't handle the pain.*

The only reason why that chiropractor allowed me to suffer for so long and withhold his knowledge about his personal success with Rolfing is as plain and simple; greed and egotism. It still bothers me that he chose to let me suffer on top of draining my insurance company. Now that insurance companies are limiting or stopping their chiropractic coverage many chiropractors will be out of business. This maybe an initial painful process but in the end only the *quality-practors* will survive.

Chiropractic care isn't the only health-related arena that can be found guilty of being close-minded. This is a danger in all health professions and both chiropractors and naturopaths alike have been guilty of not communing enough to create a holistic community of shared knowledge. The chiropractic profession has fought long and hard to get where it is today and has had to make many concessions to be taken seriously. In fact, in 1987 the American Medical Association was convicted of conspiring overtly and covertly to destroy the chiropractic profession for over twelve years. Also convicted were the American College of Surgeons and the American College of Radiologists (Ausubel, 2000). The chiropractic field is fortunate to have attained a respected status within the allopathic realm. It has, however, taken its toll within the profession, and has, perhaps, caused chiropractors to feel isolated out of fear of being "disenfranchised" again. The truth is simple: we all need to come together to share our wealth of knowledge and stop judging each other from the perspectives of biased assessment and fear.

The second reason I blame for the lack of results in methods of natural healing is the ineffectiveness of self-diagnosing. Our deepest chronic blocks are what we ourselves cannot (or refuse) to see. Here I offer an example from my own experience. Before I became a doctor of natural health I tried unsuccessfully for three years to overcome a chronic candida infection that I had been carrying for over 25 years. When I finally did get rid of it, it came right back. I had the same experience with weight gain.

This recurrence happened for two reasons. The first is that I had started self-healing because of the poor results I had attained from various local naturopaths. More importantly, I did not want to see or deal with the core emotional issues that were inevitably attached to my chronic disorder. I had a dairy addiction that stood in my way from finding wellness and whenever I attempted to

Introduction

go off of dairy I would get angry and then that anger would be followed by excuses. The excuses in my mind were always reasons why I could or should be allowed to have it.

These types of emotions kept me running in place for years. I started working with an Orgonomist doctor to help me explore and release my emotional blocks to wellness. It was within the context and treatment path of Orgonomy that I realized that milk represented my mother and could connect the potent ways that milk nurtured me both physically and emotionally. Here is a more detailed explanation of how food cravings and food related illness are directly related to childhood.

Having never been breastfed, I was given the bottle as an infant to appease my hunger for both food and maternal contact. This is because my mother had severe breast anxiety due to shaming by her own parents. Because of her inability to make "contact" emotionally with me she resorted to over feeding me instead of holding me when I cried. Chronic infant avoidance was also evidenced by having my sisters feed me in a baby chair or propping the bottle up in my crib.

Later, my father used food to punish me; I would not get any dinner if I misbehaved and I would be sent to my room. My relationship with food was even further complicated throughout my life as a young adult as it was not unusual for my father to eat off my plate, even before I was finished. In high school I remember being embarrassed when a friend came over to eat. I sat helplessly by as my father snatched up most of the food, out of a fear that we would take it from him. Thus, it became clear that he had been punished with food as well.

I spent many years bouncing back and forth between starving myself (anorexia) and binge eating accompanied by vomiting (bulimia). Overcoming these disorders including obesity only occurred when I became conscious of the reasons why and how, the core of the illness. How many people with food disorders would be helped by just becoming conscious of the fine line between food that heals and food that harms? Truly one can eat healthy food but one must also be able to accept the nourishment of that food and feel worthy enough to be nourished as well. It is a process of consciousness which is only created by our willingness to become honest and truthful about our life and feelings.

We can self-diagnose and earnestly study health and the human body, but as individuals many of us lack the ability to be honest with ourselves. We are constantly trying to lie to ourselves and others, often with the best, or at least most distracted intentions. Until, we as a society can overcome that primary dilemma; we will not be able to effectively self-cure. The mirror of ourselves is forever crowded by our childhood experiences and the truth of ourselves lies somewhere behind the often painfully distorted images.

So, let's begin this journey of self-examination and consciousness. In this book we will look at the importance of knowing who we are. All healing and health depends on this premise and needs to be considered within that light. Next, we will look at therapies that extract those qualities from our very soul and release them for healing and for the true ascension of the human race. This book is actually the third in the series of books I have written in an effort to help transform the current health crisis. In all my books, the moral is the same--the most important question we must ask ourselves honestly is not *how* we will be healed, but rather, do we really *want* to be?

Chapter 1

The Medical Kingdom and its Lowly Subjects

I spent the first few years of my career in the medical field, believing wholeheartedly that I could change it for the better. Preparing for a career in nursing, I learned about drugs, x-rays, Latin names, and shorthand. Nothing I could have learned about the functional prerequisites to nursing, however, could have prepared me for some of the stark truths I would encounter.

On the job in the medical office, I saw people dying—adults and children alike. I saw doctors and nurses lying to patients and laughing at them behind their backs. I saw too many numb, overworked and underpaid nurses. I saw an orchestrated money-making machine built to abuse and take advantage of weakened patients. Quantity and the increase of the flow of money were primary. Care, compassion, and respect for the dignity of the suffering—these are things I did not see to any great degree.

I chose to do my externship at an oncology clinic because I believed I could help cancer patients. When I witnessed the monopoly between chemotherapy and death and doctors, I felt ready to abandon my dream of becoming a nurse. One particular situation that upset me was the way x-rays were handled in the office. At school I was trained in the calculations of radiation versus body weight ratio. When I arrived at the clinic, my instructions were to give everyone the same dose (mega dose) of radiation because it took too much time to calculate the figures. This horrified me. I felt guilty every time I did it. I even questioned the head nurse about the effect of too much radiation on a cancer patient. This elicited a look of enervated shock rather than revelation or understanding. Not only did she not care about what I had to say, but I was warned I would lose my job if I did not just "do" what I was told to do. I was six inches taller than the head nurse, who had a wall of certificates of honor and recognition, but after having speaking with her, I felt I was only six inches high. I specifically remember her watching over me from then on, carefully making sure I gave an emaciated 90-pound 70-year-old woman a dose of x-ray for a person of 250 pounds. The contributions to humanity I planned to make were now senseless dreams.

After this encounter with the head nurse, I kept getting in trouble for taking "too much time" with the patients. I had to get them in and out more quickly and efficiently. Most of these patients were elderly and using walkers. I would hold their hand, get them some water or ask them how they were doing. Regardless of my individual effort, it was more like watching cattle standing in line to be slaughtered. The saddest thing was that these patients really believed—or should I say *wanted* to believe—that the doctors and nurses truly cared and were fully committed to their recovery and wellness.

My time at the oncology office finally expired when I got up enough nerve to question one of the "doctors." I noticed that several patients who were coming in for chemo lived on the same street and had non-Hodgkin's lymphoma. They were all coming in on different days, and I did not realize until later that this was arranged purposefully so they would not see each other. Alarmed, I took this information to one of the oncologists thinking, honestly, that he did not know—did not see this incredibly important connection. I said, "Doctor, don't you think we should let these patients know that they all live on the same street and have the same cancer?" This is when this doctor, this elderly, miserly "man of science" looked down on me with both tight, furrowed eyebrows joined in wrinkles of anger, pointed his long, boney finger at me within one inch of my eye and said, "We will do no such thing and it's none of your business!"

I felt like I was working for the Nazis in a death camp; the doctors were milking these patients dry before they died. I was being viewed by my "superiors" as an inferior busybody and I was getting the cold shoulder from everyone there but my dear patients. Many of them looked forward to seeing me a few times a week and would bring me cookies and little gifts. While I felt honored to be a part of their lives, it was painfully evident that the system was truly useless and utterly broken. Since my hands were tied, when my externship was over, I went to work in a pediatric clinic, hoping to be able to accomplish my dream of helping humanity there.

The pediatric clinic proved to be even more disturbing than the oncology center. Instead of older people with difficult conditions coming in the doors, there were frightened innocent children and parents who were anxious, ill-advised and seeking.

One of my jobs at the pediatric clinic was to give vaccinations to children. This was a heart-wrenching job and I quickly learned I was nothing more than a henchman for the doctor. The first thing I did not like to do was lie to the patients, saying that the doctor was in his office when he was, in fact outside, smoking. That proved to be trivial compared to what I was about to witness and experience. Vaccinating the children was a lot different than practicing with water shots at school with my fellow students. In the office I had to hold children down kicking and screaming--I had to forcefully inject them with a myriad of carcinogenic drug compounds. I quickly learned that this was the most unpleasant job there could possibly be—wasn't I supposed to be helping people? Looking into the eyes of small, beautiful, helpless babies and physically harming them is a terrible thing. In order to do it, you have to be completely and utterly convinced that what you are doing is the right thing for the well- being of the child and the community. Perhaps therein sits the root of my burgeoning problem.

The first time I saw a vaccinated child have a severe vaccine reaction and go into anaphylactic shock, I was shocked myself to find out that no one gave a damn in the office. The doctor would not (or should I say *refused* to report) the reaction or any reactions to the CDC. Furthermore, it was a known fact in our office that we had to "cover" for the doctor and drug companies. This meant that when the parents of children called our office from the hospital, we (the nurses) had to do everything in our power to convince the parents that the SIDS, encephalitis or whatever other disease manifesting from the vaccine was not because of the vaccine. I saw this happen three times. Each time, the doctor was standing next to the nurse who was on the phone, prompting her about what to say. Another time, the nurse blamed the parent for signing the consent form saying, "Well, you signed it and you are not supposed to vaccinate your child when they are sick. You know your child better than we do." It was at this point that I started to catch on that the piece of paper I was having people sign was not to help the parent become aware of the chance of a reaction--the paper was basically another loophole created for the drug companies to eschew any liability for killing and maiming children.

I was taught in school that when you give a vaccine you have to write down exactly where on the body you gave it, write down the batch number, and then initial it. This was the standard practice that was set in place in case there was a reaction. The meaning of these reports went far beyond bookkeeping—these important reports to the CDC would ensure that all vaccines from the manufacturer would be pulled and remade. The term for a vaccine that caused a reaction was a "hot batch" and upon a report of a hot batch, there was supposed to be a hot batch alert in place for the protection of American children. Unfortunately, working out in the field, this was farthest from the truth of daily practice.

The first time I ever asked the doctor to report a reaction he replied, "What reaction?" This is the same doctor who was courted extensively by the wealthy drug representatives who were always coming in an out—an endless procession. This is the same doctor who I was made to lie for over and over. More than that, I had to lie to patients and ultimately, to myself.

In this position, I was required to have the parents sign a paper saying that the chance of reaction was one out of one hundred. It also stated that the children were not to be vaccinated if they were sick with a cold or had a fever. I was instructed that if any parent protested or seemed uneasy, I was to comfort them and "convince" them that what they were doing to their children was "right." Many parents would look at me and look down at the ground, as if they were definitely not trusting and listening to their inner voice as their children were vaccinated. Some of these parents had the distinct notion that what they were doing to their child was wrong. They were looking at me, wanting to trust me, but I was representing the doctor and he was representing the drug companies. The parents were scared and they wanted to believe or they needed to believe that what they were doing was right.

Whether vaccines are "good" or "bad" for the physical body is a separate issue from even the trauma experienced by the child when the vaccine is injected. I—being a complete stranger to them--have had to hold children down with my whole body. They would be kicking, crying, screaming, and begging me to stop. We would bribe the children with candy if they would just "let us do this to them." The whole process was severely emotionally scarring and draining to everyone involved. One mother was supposed to hold a child's arms down and I was holding his legs. The woman let go of her child and the child jumped up and ripped the vaccine out of my hand and out of his leg. It was a frantic scene and I had to struggle to get it back from him. Of course, the mother blamed me for being an incompetent nurse, but looking back at my experience, she was not alone. So many parents felt uneasy about what they were doing to their children. Many looked white and pale. The idea was that they had to hurt their child to protect them; they needed someone to blame. The guilt was so great on all of us.

Inhaler Candy: They're free, Take One!

I should mention something else that bothered me while working at the pediatric clinic, the common practice of handing out asthma inhalers to sick children. I thought this practice was long gone by now, but lo and behold; a good friend of mine's daughter was given an asthma inhaler to treat a lung infection in 2007. At the time, the child's mother seemed to be relieved and thankful for the doctor's generous, free gift. That relief was short-lived, however, when I told her how dangerous it was to treat lung infections with asthma inhalers.

The practice first came to my attention in 1996. I would see drug companies come in with boxes of inhalers for the doctors to pass out. Cute and colorful, I was not immediately alarmed. A short time after, I noticed the doctor handing them out to practically every child that came in. Were these inhalers some kind of miracle lung-healing apparatuses? Of course not; because you guessed it, these, were another ploy by the drug companies to push their brands on unsuspecting health consumers.

All of this inhaler business came to a head when we received a call at the doctor's office from a mother at the hospital with a dying child. Turned out the cute, colorful inhaler became a deadly weapon in the hands of a child with pneumonia. Yes, the doctor had given the child who had pneumonia an inhaler! This caused the bronchioles to dilate and push the infection deeper and farther into the lungs. I remember the doctor getting off the phone with the sobbing mother and smugly defending himself by saying, "How was I supposed to know the kid was that sick! He didn't look that sick to me!"

The King and his Harem

At the pediatric office, I had a sick and disturbing opportunity to witness and be a part of a kind of child molestation. I say I was a part of it because at that time, I did not do anything about it and chose not to do anything about it. I had already, up until this time, seen how things that happened could make so many waves for me professionally while so few for those who were irresponsibly handling their important charges—these small children. In hindsight, I think that perhaps I was becoming exhausted with all of the numbing trickery and lies. However, I tell this story because it needs to be known and because this is my effort to educate others so that it never has to happen again. I was able to see firsthand how a highly-respected man in our culture, because of his status as wealthy and male, lets out his sexually repressed anger and hatred on unsuspecting females.

The pediatrician I worked for lived in an affluent area and was a favorite of many of the women and mothers from that community. They trusted him and he was fairly young (40s) and several mothers had joked with me about how they thought he was "good looking." I didn't. When I first started working there I would see the doctor go back and forth to a daycare center that he owned next door. I later learned that he was married to a young woman, barely twenty years old, and they had three children together. His wife, who only spoke broken English, was constantly calling and coming up to the office crying. At first I thought this girl was an insecure housewife, but I soon learned from the nurses at the office that he was indeed a cheater. He had a habit of sleeping with the women he had running the daycare center next door and with other women as well.

This doctor I worked for really loved his "respected" position. He was treated like a god; the drug companies came in and gave him beautiful trips and expensive gifts. He was used to getting what he wanted because of his title. After about two months, I finally got to see how far the line could be crossed for a respected "medical doctor."

A thirteen-year old girl came in with her mother. I took her information, weight and pulse, and ushered her into a treatment room. I was told by the other nurses that she had been a regular at the office for years. She was complaining that she was sick with a cold and was too "old" for her mom to be in the room. This elicited an exasperated, hurt look from the mother, but she immediately left the room, probably out of embarrassment. After a few minutes, the doctor went in to see her, with his "trusted" nurse and not me. Initially, I thought this was strange, since I was the one who took the girl's information, but then again, I was not a trusted nurse.

You see, at this office, to be a trusted nurse, this meant far more than being reliable and hard-working in one's duty as a nurse--this meant being a woman who would lie to his wife, the patients—lie to anyone for him and "the cause."

The doctor walked out of the room like a gleeful teenage boy who had found a porn magazine under his dad's bed. He was gloating and rubbing his hands together, pacing back and forth. He started asking for me to look for some gentian violet (which is used as a smear for microscope specimens) so he could do a vaginal exam on the young girl. I said, "Doctor, we don't have a lab here, you know we don't have any microscopes or gentian violet." This information made no impression on him whatsoever. He was dead-set on examining the girl.

"Well that's okay," he said, "I am going to check her out anyway; she told me she has been having sex with lots of guys!"

This man was now a bloodthirsty spider, drooling at the prospect of finding some helpless prey fall into his web. The unsuspecting, trusting mother sat patiently in the lobby thumbing through old magazines. The scared, fearful girl lay on her back with her legs open, believing that the trusted doctor was going to help her.

It was all too much for me. I stood outside the room and started pacing back and forth myself. The other patients, the files and charts—all of those ordinary elements of daily life as a nurse were far from my mind. What I wanted to do was rescue that girl, go in to that room and stop that doctor/man from having his way with her.

After several moments passed, the doctor emerged from the room, strutting like a proud peacock—work finished, mission accomplished, "kudos" given. He went on to tell all of the nurses in the back, "What a slut, what a whore, that vagina was so sickening, she must have had sex with every guy she saw! She's gotta have like gonorrhea or syphilis or something."

The nurses cackled. Sitting high on their cloud of moral condemnation, they reveled in the doctor's details. The nurses at any clinic I worked at always reminded me of the applause and laughter button that gets pushed in a sitcom whenever someone makes a joke, funny or not. They would blindly follow and support this man for every diabolical, incomprehensible, lascivious move he made. This was all, of course, at less than one-quarter of the doctor's wage.

Meanwhile, a mere twenty feet from where the doctor stood, the young girl was getting dressed in the "treatment room." She had yet again been used and abused by someone she trusted. The doctor walked into the waiting room, looked at the mother in the eyes and blatantly lied to her. He effectively covered for the girl and also for himself. He told her he was prescribing some antibiotics for the cold and did not mention the vaginal exam or suspicion of STDs. The mother asked no questions and as I recall, thanked him more than once. They disappeared from the office, but never has that young girl disappeared from my heart.

How often do these things happen? Well, you might think this is an isolated incident. But to be honest with you this subject hits close to home as I was abused myself as a teenager by an untrustworthy doctor. My first gynecological exam turned into a hellish nightmare of black mail and shame. My boyfriend (who is now my husband) and I were using latex condoms to have sex. I soon developed an infection, in which I carefully described to my mother as a "yeast infection" as I had not confided in her that I was having sex. This is where all of my problems began.

My mother took me to a female gynecologist who was a small frail looking Indian woman. She was very kind to me in front of my mother and I too requested my mother to leave the room as I was "too old" and embarrassed. Alone with the doctor she grilled me about having sex, she made me feel bad, alone and ashamed. She used a harsh tone with me and even made references to me being an American and a slut. After the shame session she examined me and concluded I had a latex allergy.

Now here are the parts that are questionable and even torturous. She agreed to lie to my mom to get me on birth control pills by convincing my mother that I was having problems with menstruation. Secondly, she prescribed antibiotics for the infection.

Thirdly, and most shockingly, she recommended not only a pap smear but tissue samples and cryosurgery for my cervix. I was told that my pap smear was irregular. For this or for the sex, I was "punished" severely.

The pap smear was unusually painful and crampy. Then came the tissue samples, in which she inserted a tool that looked like a hole puncher and removed parts of my cervix. At this I started crying, I was then told I better not cry and if I did she would tell my mother that I had been having sex. So, I sucked in the pain and abuse. A week after the tissue sampling came the cryosurgery. Where she literally froze and sloughed off all of the tissue on my cervix. The pain I felt during that month caused a residual damage to my emotions and psyche that would reappear ten years later in the problems I had delivering my children. The theme of non-progression, long labor and an inability to cry or scream during labor was present during each labor and delivery.

Regardless of personal moralistic views pertaining to teenage girls and sex, every girl deserves to be loved, guided and protected during medical treatment. Often, the people who have an opportunity to help the teenager either misses the opportunity, closes their eyes to it or consciously ignores it. I also don't think I would be exaggerating by concluding that there is a passive aggressive anger in the treatment of the teenagers. A type of sadistic happiness that the girl is getting what she deserves. This is when it all becomes a cultural circle of abuse, where everyone in our society takes a turn preying on the weak, sick, and underprivileged.

I've seen it with girls raised in strict moral and religious families and I have also seen it in "quasi" religious families where laissez-faire parents still hold the same puritanical prejudices as fundamental families. Neither one of these systems are giving young girls what they need and neither one is working. The latter needs to give love and guidance and the first needs to give freedom and acceptance. Putting most of the responsibility on the mother still doesn't let a doctor abusing his position off the hook. We need to realize that what we hide or do not want to look at honestly as parents, are obvious to those around us, especially predators.

This is not to say that every oncology doctor out there is a cold, narcissistic, sadist. I also do not wish to imply that every pediatrician is a womanizing, pedophile and that health-care that cares does not exist. To the contrary, I believe if you have a good doctor, then you are lucky and should protect that relationship with your patients at all costs. With that being said, it is still, utterly important that, as a society, we take a look at the other side of health care. The side that you may not see or experience in the waiting room or fifteen-minute office visit. I only ask that we all thoughtfully examine the care we are receiving through the medical establishment. Have we been ignoring our better judgment and intuition in some circumstances? Have we been willingly but unknowingly putting ourselves or our children in harms way? This brings us to another question, who do we trust and why do we trust them?

Don't Talk to Strangers....

We are experiencing a generationally-conditioned response within this country by which parents have willingly allowed strangers to hold their children down and inject them with vaccines, to remove sections of the most sensitive and important parts of the body (as with circumcision), and even to watch over their children. I attribute this to the fact that many people in this culture, including me, have been raised in puritan-inspired homes. The idea has been sold to us that there are "special" people out there who know more about God than we do, more about children than we do, and more about health than we do. Clearly, we have been led to believe, against our better judgment, that we must blindly follow and respect people who do not deserve our respect. The ability to effectively think for ourselves has been greatly impaired and the people who know that abuse that premise.

There are certain biblical tenants that are the hallmark of our Judeo-Christian country. Some of them are "Spare the rod, spoil the child" and "A Father that loves his children, chastises them." Beliefs like these have had a detrimental effect on society as a whole.

Although was raised Catholic, I left the Catholic Church for 20 years to study different denominations of Christianity and religions such as Judaism and Hinduism. I worshipped with Baptists, Reformists (Calvinists), Non-Denominationalists, and Messianic-Jews, I even took Hebrew and recited the prayer "Baruch ata Adonai, Eloheinu, Melech ha Olam" every day. These experiences also led me to write a separate book on this, as religion continues to fascinate me. As I look back at all of my experiences, I remember sermons at a Baptist church that encouraged people to abuse and hurt their children. The message is often or sometimes, "If you don't hit your children, you don't love them."

One would not be blasphemous to admit there are some contradictions in the Bible, indicating a contrast between "good and bad." Although life itself is both an internal and external yin and yang, opposing forces, in this case, it has created a type religious/emotional chaos. For some reason, people rectify these contradictions by thinking they are following the good while overwhelming producing actions that coincide with the bad. In some instances of Biblical texts, specifically the ones which are the direct quotes of Jesus, we find a loving and accepting God who also loves children and heals the masses equally.

However in the Old Testament there are recommendations for male infant genital mutilation (circumcision) and a story about God where he even abuses and kills little children himself. (2 Kings 2:24, the story of Elisha with the children). While many people seem to gloss over these aspects of the Bible, these beliefs are heavily cemented in our society and are a monumental burden on our children and our children's children.

Because the deeper softer emotions of love and healing are so difficult and far from Western psyche, the harsher and more pain inducing aspects are often easier to follow. We might describe this as Christians having not integrated New Testament teaching into their lives and families. While I don't mean to exclude other religions, the truth is every person would be prudent to come to terms with the contradictions in their own religions and make conscious decisions on which side they are on.

I was raised in a home where I was spanked. This was directly attributed to my parent's belief that children are born as product of sin and need to be "made" as good. I was subjected to bizarre and confusing rituals as a child growing up in a Catholic home. I call them bizarre and confusing, given my age and my inability to understand the purpose and meaning behind them. One in particular, reconciliation, was frightening to me.

I was sent into a room alone with a strange man (the Priest) that I was scared of and didn't know. Then, I was told by my parents and teachers to tell this man about everything I had done wrong in order to be forgiven. I came out of the room both shaking and with a sigh of relief. I looked into the sea of faceless faces and saw my family looking at me joyful and with pride. I was even given a party and lots of money from relatives for going through with that terrifying ordeal.

As an adult, I now have come to appreciate the rituals and religion I was brought up with. It is my opinion that if my parents had waited until I was older and even let me choose to make my sacraments it would have been a better experience for me as a whole. I now see this in my own children who did not become baptized or make their Catholic sacraments until they showed interest and were old enough to understand. In this way they were considered converts and were eleven and ten years old. Even though I had harsh views about the Church and religion in general, it was the gentle love and faith of my children which softened my heart and brought me to a balanced place in my life.

How Health Care Affects the Children

Regardless of the positive and negative consequences of religion, one must always seek to maintain balance. As it stands, many nonsensical and horrendous beliefs about children form the backbone of our society. Even if we do not hit and spank our children, many of us still participate in practices destructive to children's mental health that are not overtly religious in nature or origin. At what age were *we* lead by the hand to a medical priesthood that did not deserve our trust and our hard-earned dollars? What medical system deserves the blood sacrifice of our children's lives? We first allow heartless, hardened doctors of medicine, into our innermost sanctum, our births. Then we hand our beloved babies and children over to them, thoughtlessly, over and over throughout their lives. We tell our children not to go with strangers but what kind of example are we setting?

I apologize if it seems that I am being unfair to the many good medical, chiropractic, and naturopathic professionals out there. The truth is that many people in this world are contributing positively to humanity just by having good intentions and not necessarily all of the answers. My focus is on the grave underworld that is affecting this country, the people who live for profit, the heartbeat of capitalism that has affected all of us (in good and bad ways). Weakness or sickness in our country means money and profit for others. Salesmen and advertisements are also a part of this scheme. Simply put, if someone is not in their right mind and in good health, they are food for the greedy wolves with stomachs that can never be filled. We can see this in nature, when other animals come upon one that is sick and weakened; they often tear it limb from limb and devour it.

Darwin's Contribution to Health and Healing

This brings me to how Darwin's survival of the fittest, which coincides completely with religion, racism, and classism, and has a lot to do with our present state of crisis. In the book *The Dark Side of Christian History*, author Helen Ellerbe asserts that while Christianity and Darwinism appear to be foes, that they are actually two sides of the same coin. The only reason why Darwinism was allowed to go as far as it did was because it fed the idea that one is always better or more important than another. Darwin's theory fits in perfectly with all political structures: socialism, capitalism, fascism and even communism. Only the most powerful, privileged, and richest people are at the top-- the rest of us are merely licking up the scraps. This mindset has allowed some of us to believe we do not deserve to be happy, healthy, and wealthy. Is it sin that keeps us in our present state of disease, or is it simply a decrepit belief system passed down from generation to generation, from mother to child, child to adulthood, from adulthood to the entire world? In my other books I delve more deeply into maternal belief systems and their effects on the fetus and society as a whole.

Your health and life are compromised and changed as a result of creationist or evolutionist theories. These ideas assert that it is they who are better, stronger, and more powerful than I. The hole in our heart is created by fanatical dogma a paradigm that tells us that we are depraved. It tells us we should be continually looking for God's parental approval. This is hole that we can attempt to have filled by drugs (yes, prescription drugs are drugs!), addictions, sickness and fanatical religious groups. One aspect that would propel us onto the road toward healing our entire society is simply changing our beliefs about ourselves. The truth is that we all have the "divine" right and ability to heal ourselves, or as Christ would say, "The kingdom of God is within us."

The Body - Mind Connection

> *"Through the millennia, humanity has more or less consciously known that all diseases ultimately have a psychic origin and it became a "scientific" asset firmly anchored in the inheritance of universal knowledge; it is only modern medicine that has turned our animated beings into a bag full of chemical formulas."*
>
> *Dr. Ryke Geerd Hamer.*

Dr. R.G. Hamer of Germany, in observing over ten thousand cases of cancer patients, found that cancer, heart diseases, and many other illnesses are triggered by emotional factors. Often a combination of shock, or conflict and not being able to talk about it will produce lesions in the brain within a few months (Hamer, 2008). Dr. Valerie Hunt, in nearly thirty years of laboratory research, has found that human energy fields are related to thoughts and emotions (Hunt, 2009). Psychics are able to observe changes in this energy in the color of the field or aura of the human body.

It is no longer an issue about whether or not the mind-body connection is necessary for healing—this is a proven fact. The real dilemma we face is this: what emotional obstacles do we need to overcome so that health can effectively overcome sickness in the body? We know the mind can heal the body, but what if the mind is clouded, confused, or depressed? What if there is an attempt in the mind to heal the body but it is continually thwarted and diverted by repressed issues and trauma stored deep within the system? We can think and think ourselves to better health, but in the end all of us are subject to the pain and problems we refuse to face.

Feelings and emotions are the most important and yet most filtered and repressed aspects of our personality. Many of us are continually diverting dimensions of our true selves. It as if our feelings come up from deep within us and meet road blocks and detour after detour. Oh, we think we know how we feel, but often we express the opposite. I catch myself doing it all the time, wanting to express love to someone, but finding it comes out as hate. Feeling hate, I therefore express love at the physical surface only. I find myself continually fighting to express and find my true feelings. Wilhelm Reich, the founder of Orgonomy and discoverer of orgone energy, is the only researcher I have found that has stood up for the true expression of human emotion. Even Valerie Hunt's important research on emotions and bioenergy totally misses the mark when she recommends "escaping" reality through hypnotism or mysticism to cure chronic disease. While I do not assert that these methods are not effective on various levels, the important issue at hand is; how long can we run and hide from ourselves before our true self catches up to us? We cannot and hide and when we do, we merely manifest other new physical symptoms from time to time in the form of anxiety disorders, headaches, breathings difficulties, etc. Many who have unsuccessfully tried to mystically recreate or change their personalities with magic words and affirmations know exactly what I am talking about.

Health then, becomes more than just mind over matter—it is a matter of truth and reality over lies and deception. Some people like to use trendy, pretty language to describe the road to wellness, such as declaring that stress causes illness and compassion and forgiveness are necessary components of health. All of those words are merely symptoms and smokescreens for the real problem, which is emotional repression. Let us look at the negative emotions for what they are: hatred, anger and contempt. The very act of tiptoeing around uncomfortable words only enables people to shrink farther and farther away from their true feelings. We are taught not to trust our feelings in this society, but I assure you, find someone's true feelings and you find the most important piece in the puzzle of sickness.

Faith-Based Healing

Bringing the body and mind together is much more difficult than it seems. Religion tells people to bring their sickness to God; then it tells them they are bad and to ask for forgiveness; and *then* it tells them to bring it back to God again when it does not work. This is not to imply that faith healing doesn't work, but when we moralize sickness, the sick person believes they are bad and that they are being punished for their sins. This mindset does little to heal the body and even less for their spiritual relationship with God. One precept of Christian teaching is that the wages of sin is death. Some churches will tell you that your only hope, then, is to rely on Jesus to forgive you and heal you. This leads us to the question, what exactly is our perception of Jesus?

As a Christian I thought of Jesus not as the loving, accepting figure he says he is in the red letters of the Bible, but as the mean, crazed, angry man he is portrayed as in the book of Revelations (a book that contradicts all prior teachings about Jesus in the Bible). I thought of God as in the "Santa Claus is Comin' to Town" song. He saw me when I was sleeping, he knew when I was awake and he knew if I was bad or good. I was always personally afraid of him as a child. Here was a man I had never seen, who was supposed to be everywhere and who was watching me at all times. Even within the context of Jesus, I was taught that Jesus loved me and all the little children, but the overwhelming message I received was that I was a bad girl and was going to be punished for my sins. We can all see how that type of belief system affects our health and well-being. With such belief systems driven with stakes at birth into our being, can we be surprised when hypnotic affirmations are not enough to convince us otherwise?

I use Christianity as an example because that was the religion I was raised within; surely, you can apply this same situation to any religion and faith-based mindset.

Mystical Affirmations: Just Love.....

Even the new-age sector, where new-agers often pride themselves on loving and accepting others unconditionally, has missed the mark on healing in certain ways. Some new age practices are teaching people to just "tell themselves" that they are love, peace or health. While I wouldn't argue that these practices are not helping somewhat through self-hypnosis, in the long-term, these practices are simply not enough to break severe physical and emotional constraints that have been plaguing the body and mind for an entire lifetime. I give a terrific example of this phenomena in chapter four.

The traumas that many of us hold in our body are often cemented into our heads as children through a variety of reinforcements, whether in the physical form of slaps or beatings, or the less overt, which might include simply a look of hatred from the parental figure to the child. The act of rejection from parent to child for not living up to the parent's expectations is far more commonplace than it seems. Please keep in mind the "perception" the child has, and to a child, the parent is literally "God" to the child. Most children are born to continually seek parental acceptance and to be continually let down in that aspect.

I often think the of the greatness that would become manifest in our society were it the other way around, with children being born into love and fully accepted for the truth of who they are and who they will be. How can our children ever be given a chance at "themselves", when we are always projecting our own inadequacies and emotional baggage onto them? We can never know the pure and "un-adulterated" nature of the human personality, but we can certainly try our hardest to help our children get there.

Chapter 2

Healing the Body, Healing the Mind

The Medical Exodus

The final blow to my dream of becoming a nurse occurred when I called the local news station, thinking yet again that I was doing something to help humanity.

One morning at 9 a.m., while watching TV, I saw a news reporter urging people to tune in that night for the 6 o'clock news to see the story of how the hepatitis B vaccine is linked to childhood arthritis. There were pictures on the screen of several children that were sick and injured from the vaccine. I could not believe my eyes—could not believe something like that could be true and moreover, that it would garner the media attention it deserved. Are they really going to blow the cover off this mass deception?

I, like the naïve, optimistic young woman I was, actually called the news station. I talked to the reporter and told her that I used to work as a nurse in a local doctor's office that administered vaccines and that I had witnessed many unreported reactions. She said, "Would you be willing to go on TV and tell your story?" I said, "Of course!" She then asked for the names of any doctors I knew that were against the vaccine and I gave her the name and number of one that I personally knew and trusted. She said, "Great, we will be at your house for an interview in an hour."

By 11 a.m. I had TV cameras and reporters crowding into my house. I invited my sister to come over to see the commotion. We could not believe what was happening. When the news reporter got there, she said that their phone had been ringing off the hook for weeks regarding reactions to vaccinations. Apparently, some parents were actually able to see through the vaccine propaganda and were putting some pieces together. She said parents were blaming the vaccine for arthritis, childhood diabetes, and SIDS. She told me that my interview was crucial. Then she told me that the doctor that I had recommended for them to call had refused to talk to them.

I thought that was odd because I knew this doctor and trusted him more than I trusted these reporters. Immediately, a red flag went up in my head. I started to feel afraid of what I may have done by letting these people into my home, letting them see my face and know my name.

It was at this time when we sat down to do the interview that I asked to remain anonymous and have my face darkened. The reporter agreed and started asking me a series of questions on camera. One thing I remember saying clearly was, "Even if the chance of a reaction is truly one out of a hundred, well then, as far as I am concerned, that is one too many. All children need to be protected and more research needs to be done to make these drugs safe." After the interview the media gathered their things and headed out as quickly as they had come.

My sister and I waited patiently for the 6 o'clock news to come on. Finally, when it did, a sort of terror, which I can only describe as a sickness and a burning pain in the back of my neck, came bursting down through my body. The news reporter was sitting at her desk on TV and said, "We are sorry for the confusion about the hepatitis B vaccine. We have doctors in our studio taking your calls at this moment. The doctors have reassured us that there is nothing wrong with the vaccines and they are worried people may stop vaccinating their children and stop protecting their children against this deadly disease." Then, as if that was not enough, they flashed my interview on the screen. There I was in the form of a dark shadow saying, "Reactions are only one out of a hundred."

I could not believe it! I was actually frightened for my life at that time. I felt my world come down around me. I lost all sense of trust and understanding of the world around me. I saw a grossly orchestrated effort of the entire community to make people sick and furthermore, to hurt children, for profit. Furthermore, I was experiencing, intense guilt and hate towards myself for participating in such a cold, hardened disrespect for human life. I felt betrayed and humiliated by everything I believed in.

Hope in Crisis

It was at this same time that I settled down to have children and raise a family, but I could not rest or give up on my original commitment to seek healing and health for others. Then about ten years ago, I began an intense study of Orgonomy, which developed into an intense passion and interest as I began studying how emotional trauma was held within the physical body. I have always studied this along with my Doctor of Natural Health program, and have viewed everything within that light. In that context, I read the work of the late Wilhelm Reich, Ida Rolf and also about Dr. Upledger's work on the somato- emotional release. This led me to want to see my own chronic health/ mind conditions and seek therapy for myself.

I was obsessed with this information as a whole or continuum. Viewing all sickness as an ancient thread of global proportions, I had to unearth every reason, every cause, never being satisfied, testing and retesting. Any friend or acquaintance I knew who was not feeling well was questioned and studied like an object under a magnifying glass. I made an effort to speak honestly with people about their health and found honesty was not tolerated well. Most people keep within their "dis-ease" or illness an aspect of their personality that they refuse to look at or deal with. The body keeps manifesting symptoms and deteriorating, while the person denies the help they know they need on different, often subtle levels.

Addicted to Alternative Healing and Health

There are many different levels that appear in people who refuse to deal with their illness and who ignore symptoms out of a severe lack of conscious awareness. The most subtle aspects of this lies in the way that people seek out every doctor or healing therapy available and appear to be earnestly searching for help or a cure, yet, in reality, all the effort is part of a mask. They know what they need to do, and have probably heard it already from more than one M.D. or Naturopath. When these people finally hit that wall, instead of facing the truth, they merely reroute their journey, discrediting or blaming the therapy or practitioner and moving on to something else. In my experience as a natural health doctor, I have seen more people choosing this course of action than any other.

These types of people have reached the point of consciously realizing that their body is not well, but they have yet to grasp the idea that their mindset is not. They come to me wanting an expensive herb or something that will "placate" them for a while. When I tell them a simple cost-effective treatment that involves little or no herbs, they often cry out for the magic pill/herb to remove their illness. Most of these herbs will nudge the disorder toward a more balanced state but what is required for the actual state of health is a tremendous step forward in a different direction. In short, what is required is literally a change of heart. Many want to heal the body but instead, hold on for dear life to their emotional pain.

Does it Have to Hurt to Help?

I should mention another type: the masochistic naturalist. These people are type A about health and are radically into alternative treatments. They starve their body, they go on long fasts, and they will detox, detox, and detox until their health is diminished and they feel worse. These types will not attribute their present state of feeling poorly to the radical measures they have taken in their attempts to be healed, but they will view it as evidence that they need to ravage their body more. They view their body as a war zone and in some ways want to hurt their body out of repressed anger or fear. They believe--point blank, "no pain, no gain." Some American doctors in alternative medicine support this trend of "shocking" the body into health.

It is the flipside of merely placating the disorder, bringing it to the other side of the spectrum, tearing the body apart to get to the virus/bacteria inside. In some ways it coincides with our Judeo-Christian morals that suggest the body is dirty and that suffering is good.

All of these responses and reactions are normal (although not natural) and are to be expected in a society like our own. When I was a small girl and was ill, my mother would run me off to the doctors in a fretful, weakened state herself. The common cold was another trip to the medical doctor for yet another antibiotic; month after month it was the same thing form the time I was born. My mother never understood or felt any positive response to the human body. Sickness was feared and had to be eradicated. I would look to my mother, wanting her to help me in my illness, and she would look to the doctor. Instead of preventing sickness through diet, sickness was thought to be prevented by vaccine and covered up by drugs.

My experience, as well as the experiences of others, shows how so many of us were conditioned to believe that we could not heal ourselves and were thus left in the dark when it came to the true nature of the human body. We are now (hopefully) coming out of the dark ages and entering a time where our faith will not be committed to the religious and medical hierarchy, but toward ourselves. There was a long period of time when people were killed if they looked to the anything outside of the church for healing. It was women who had the knowledge of herbs and healing and these women passed it on through a quiet, personal brand of education that got the brunt of the blame. The dark ages were a time when millions of women accused of witchcraft were killed. Their crime was simply the knowledge of the earth and herbalism; this included herbal contraception and helping women in childbirth through midwifery.

Among the darkest episodes in humanity were the periods from roughly 1300 to the 1700s. This was when there was a systematic and violent attempt to eradicate herbalism and folk medicine completely. Being an herbalist would most certainly get you accused of witchcraft, and what attributed to the hysteria were the patriarchal religious views about women in general. Shocking quotes from early founders of the Christian church such as; "every woman should be filled with shame by the thought that she is a woman." and "Let [women] die in childbirth- that is why they are there" are not hard to find (Ellerbe, 1999).

Wiping out witchcraft/herbalism was not an easy feat. It took hundreds of years and was accomplished through force, torture and even death. Looking at the long line throughout history that has been drawn against natural healing and helping ourselves, one can see how hard it is to change cultural views that have taught us not to think for ourselves, but merely to trust in someone else blindly. How convenient, to try to deem anyone trying to heal themselves outside the power of religion or medical establishment as being a Satanist or a quack. Now, just like throughout much of Western history, people are simply making money off of our ignorance and shame. Please see the reference page for recommended books if this subject interests you.

Orgonomy, What It Is, What It Isn't

In this book I attempt to simplify what it is as a means to create what we can consider to be the first rung on the ladder of conscious healing. I did not want to just write a book on Orgonomy, in part because there are many excellent books already written on the subject. My two favorites are *Emotional Armoring: an Introduction to Psychiatric Orgone Therapy* by Morton Herskowitz and *Saharasia* by James DeMeo.

So what is Orgonomy exactly? Orgonomy is the study of orgone energy (ether, prana, chi) and its relation to the human body and to the planet. When someone goes through orgone therapy, he or she is attempting to free up energy blocks in the body, which in turn grants greater access to energy movement through out the body. Once the energy moves through you, you "see' more clearly, you "act" more clearly, you "feel" more clearly. An Orgonomist is a medical doctor or doctor of osteopathy and has to go through years of school to even qualify for entrance into the American College of Orgonomy. These individuals are then trained to recognize body symptoms, character structure and armors which are defensive behavioral blocks.

It is a complex, ethereal process to describe, even after having experienced the therapy myself. I can only say that before the therapy I was denying that many things in my life bothered me; in fact, I was such a "laid-back" person that I seldom became angry or upset. However, there were people in my life I thought I had forgiven, but then I discovered that my perception of being laid-back was just another conditioned response. In truth, my chronic health problems were inherently connected to the emotional pain I was carrying with me from various stages of my life. The therapy unpeeled my life and ego in layers, like an onion. In some sessions I would go back to the first year of my life, in others I would go back only as far as five years. I was holding many experiences in my body, but the experiences were neither good nor bad, they just existed—they were only held in my body because of my perception of them.

In Orgonomy, you unearth surprisingly painful things and realize that nearly everything is about perception. For instance, to describe the issue of perception, consider this common scenario: you are walking into a store and the person in front of you does not see you and shuts the door on you. This happens often, but we so often do not think fully about what just transpired. What do you do when this happens? Some people think "oh, they must not have seen me" while others take it personally and will feel attacked; they may actually say something to the person (and usually not in a friendly way). Still others won't do anything physically, but inside they process that information according to their life experiences and hold on to it. To their perception, having that door shut on them may have been racially motivated or it exists as part of a grander scheme of bad experiences within the computer of their brain. Some people will talk about the person who shut the door on them for a few days or more, while some will go take their miserable feelings out on their pet, child or spouse.

While our culture is just beginning to understand crucial aspects of perception and how pain is held in the body, it has really been missing the mark when it comes to how to treat it. Too many therapies and books focus on perception and recommend one: "just forgive," or we hear recommendations like this one, "change your mind and change the experience". Are any of these powerful enough to actually address the issue of perception or do they all recommend "quick fixes" for matters that go far beyond the event itself?

Orgone therapy provides a different way to respond and perceive these issues. It is one of the few treatments that says, "No, it's not okay to carry this around, stop lying to yourself, you need to get it out of your body!" This is what makes Orgonomy unique--it *physically* takes emotional pain out of the body. I spent years in counseling, with psychologists, priests, pastors and even psychics and found that all of the talking and all of the "bullshit" was unnecessary. All I needed to do was see it and open myself up enough to let it out. While it seems simple, when practiced, for most of us at least due to our current perceptions, it is not. We are so busy trying to run the marathon so that we can get away from ourselves (and we honestly believe we will cross the finish line at some point), that to really look at ourselves honestly is unpleasant for almost all of us, and quite impossible for others.

The focus of Orgonomy is on examining energy blockages in segments of the human body. The segments start from the top of the head and continue to the pelvis. In my experience with Orgone treatment, when one segment was opened, another became blocked. Even in Naturopathy an emotional/physical block is hard to miss. For instance, someone with chronic sinus congestion, allergies, itchy watery eyes and headaches, who cannot make eye contact and wears glasses, is very likely someone who could be holding a lot in their ocular segment (behind the eyes). While I am not an Orgonomist doctor, in my natural health practice I process this information and treat or refer them accordingly. While I will; get more into treatment in my subsequent chapters, these are some important basics that required introduction.

Help is on the Way

I had to get on a plane and travel across three states to see an Orgonomist doctor. For the masses of people who could derive great benefit from this therapy, there should be something that provides in-between treatment. The therapy I offer is what I consider to be a close second to Orgonomy. I hope to *lead* people to Reich's information and Orgone therapy rather than try to replace it. I consider it as one of the first rungs on the ladder toward self-realization.

For those of you who know something about Orgonomy, you are probably familiar with bioenergetics. This is a therapy is considered by some to be a "gentler" form of Orgonomy, but nothing could be further from the truth. Bioenergetics has movements and exercises but it is missing the intention and thought. Bioenergetics attempts to tiptoe around the blocks and free them up without the important step of emotional connection to the pain. It lacks the essential element of "feeling" that serves as a crucial foundation for future healing. Bioenergetics is most advantageously used on infants who lack the depth and range of experiences that have created our personalities, conditioned our responses, and have ultimately led to blockages. To provide a backdrop to better understand Orgonomy, I offer you a few personal examples to highlight the ways it functions and how (and who) it can help.

I have always had chronic, "weak" lungs. This idea of having weak lungs was cemented into my head early simply by the power of suggestion. As a child, my mother would tell me, "You just have weak lungs and always will." My childhood and early adulthood were filled with many trips to the ER and doctor's office. It started out as chronic bronchitis and pneumonia, and then escalated years later into asthma. It seemed that every virus or bacteria in the air would land in my lungs but somehow not affect anyone else in my home. I got used to different drugs and breathing apparatus and of course, cough medicines and antibiotics. I later noticed how stress exacerbated my symptoms; I started to actually see how my weak lungs were becoming somewhat psychosomatic--my body was crying out, not with tears, but with wheezing, shaking, and shortness of breath.

When I went (and still go) for my Orgone treatments years ago, one thing I noticed was my lungs giving way to the breath. Before going for the treatments I had always worn a size 34 bra; when I was nursing my children it went up a little bit for a few months, but always returned to 34. Starting with treatments at a 34, I remember actually starting to tug at my bra and feeling uncomfortable before finally just taking it off. After a month or two of treatments, I went and got measured for a new bra. Lo and behold, I had gone up to a 36! In that relatively short span of time, my rib cage had expanded significantly in conjunction with my treatments. My breathing before Orgonomy was shallow and remained primarily in my stomach region. After Orgonomy, I actually started to see my chest rise and fall with my breath. I realized that my chest had been severely restricted do to severe childhood trauma and I had been holding a lot of emotional pain and fear there my entire life.

Clearly, the benefits were powerful from almost the beginning of the process of understanding and realization occurred. I am currently undergoing Rolfing treatments and I relate it loosely to Orgonomy, however there is no focus on emotional contact. Emotional contact is necessary for healing.

Parents and Their Contributions to the Chronic

In my practice as an ayurvedic doctor of natural health I try to come up with a number to define the degree of how much I feel an illness is psychosomatically-induced. This determines whether my treatments will rely heavily on herbs and homeopathy or whether I will utilize the "Aurore Method" (explained in a later chapter). My experiences have included treating women and their children for psychosomatic illness and as you can imagine, I have garnered a significant amount of practical wisdom through these experiences.

One woman came to me complaining that the doctor wanted to take out her daughter's tonsils and she wanted to save them, if she could. Her seven-year-old daughter was manifesting chronic throat infections and her breathing was somewhat compromised at night because of an enlarged uvula. I came to her home to observe her child in her environment. I recommended a few herbs but more importantly, I could see her daughter's condition was clearly more emotional than physical.

Upon examining her daughter, I noticed when she spoke that she had a slight speech impediment. Her voice actually communicated a child much younger than seven and she appeared to be shy and timid. When I asked her what was going on with her life and if there were problems at school, she spoke of some boys that were pushing her around and being mean to her. Even though this little girl had two older brothers, she definitely exhibited a marked fear of the male gender in general. I gave her a pillow and told her to hit it and scream. At first, she started laughing and giggling and couldn't scream, then I tried to play a game with her to see how loud she could scream—and she couldn't scream at all. She simply giggled and hit the pillow lightly with an open back hand.

I could see, quite obviously, that she suffered from an inability to communicate her feelings, she is and what she wants, effectively. Her anger from being bullied at school, and perhaps at home by a dominant male figure (the father was an intimidating one), was manifesting in the physical. I did some craniosacral therapy on her for over an hour. I spent a total of three hours at her home treating her and speaking with her mother, to whom I spoke candidly with. I told her that the most important thing for her daughter to do right now is to start screaming--literally finding her voice. I told the mother to work with her hitting the pillow and screaming out her frustrations, be it because of school or home. I also wrote down specific recommendations involving herbs and a certain brand of strong probiotics because the child had been on long term use of antibiotics.

I called two weeks later to check on the child's progress. The mother appeared to be agitated and barked at me, "Nothing you did worked!" Then I started to question her, "Did you get the probiotics I recommended?" She replied, "No, I didn't, I bought some of these little candy gummi bears that were cheaper." Then I asked if she had bought the raw honey and lemon I had recommended and she again replied, "No, I forgot." Finally, I asked if she was working with her daughter on the suggested screaming and hitting of a pillow, and again the answer, "No, I don't have time." I was agitated beyond words; this mother, as much as she loved her daughter and as sincere as she was about saving her daughter's tonsils, did not invest any time herself to help heal her daughter. This story is only one of many and the point is, many times it is the *parents* who are keeping the child from their deserved wellness. In this case, the mother was blaming me because she could not blame herself...and the cycle of chronic sickness and karma continues.

A Case of ADD

Another client I had called me one year after being initially seen for a short time before that. She was asking me to recommend an herbal replacement for the ADD drug her 14-year-old daughter was on. I, in good conscience, had a hard time with her request. I had spoken with the woman the year before when I had a three-hour home appointment with her and had been completely honest with her about her daughter's condition. Upon observing her daughter previously, I could detect that she had all of the symptoms of a block in her eye segment. The mother also complained of her daughter's sense of balance, telling me that the girl was clumsy and always tripping.

This 14-year-old, like the seven-year-old in my previous example, presented behavior that was associated with that of a younger person than was appropriate for her true age. She spoke in a continually whiny voice and when she spoke to her mother (even though she was much taller than her mother) she cowered, her head lowered, avoided eye contact and minced her words. She appeared to be both angry with and afraid of her mother.

Although this girl was not under my care, the mother asked me on my way out about her ADD symptoms. I mentioned that I had noticed some aspects of her behavior that were parallel to ADD symptomatically and offered a few easy instructions for things she could do. I also told her that her daughter was obviously angry and afraid of her and that she needed to let the daughter begin to express her anger and feelings. My thought was that the mother could create a safe environment for the daughter and let her know that nothing the daughter might say could cause her to stop loving her.

To help guide the healing process, I recommended the book *Holding Time* by Martha G. Welch and Mary Ellen Mark and said that I would see the two together to help them work it out. I should mention that although my recommendations seem to be easy to follow, I often see my clients and their children a few times together to get them started, although in the case, the process did not work according to that schedule. At that time, I also recommended an Orgonomist that would help her daughter work out and begin to address her problems.

Instead of receiving an open response, the mother, who was a fundamentalist Christian, started carrying on about evil spirits, praying, and God. I left there knowing that there would be little chance that the mother would call me or the Orgonomist to help her and her daughter. Her fundamental belief system caused her to dismiss her daughter's behavior as a cry for the mother's help. She had failed to see the real problem, which was as simple as a daughter's need to re-bond and connect with her. In this case, only the mother held the answer to whether the child would be helped and healed. The daughter was getting some attention with her behavior on some level, but it would take an orchestrated effort on her mother's part to truly help her child. Being honest with herself and her daughter would be the first step.

As the saying goes, you can lead a horse to water but you cannot make it drink. The mother quite possibly spent the entire year praying and talking about her problems with her church group. Many times these types of groups will foster and perpetuate specific religious beliefs that actually keep people from approaching the problem honestly and getting the help they need. For example, someone in the group may realize they are a child abuser and openly admit their sin. Others in the group may play down the admittance by showing the person verses in the Bible that "prove" child abuse is acceptable. Now the person returns home, confident that they are serving God in what they choose to do as an abuser, they may no longer question themselves from within.

I can attest firsthand to this phenomenon. This may come as a surprise given some of the discussions about religious fervor and self-realization that have already been presented, but I spent many years as a born-again Christian. I can tell you; the power of the peer group is quite overwhelming. Many people in religious groups are suffering emotionally and they also tend to be people who respond to fear because so much of their lives are based on fear. While they confess to have found god and the "answer", they continually seek to be validated and accepted by that god in whatever way they can. When these seekers converge in a group, instead of truly helping each other to self-realize, they end up proliferating old wives' tales and rumors, in the name of god and under the guise of godliness. Typically, their stories are based on someone who knew someone and they will often serve the sinful life circumstances of a personal friend on a plate to each other.

A conversation may begin with valid concerns about everyday problems; children, teenagers and spouses acting out their rejection and pain. The group will open up and even pray, but then the subject almost always takes an inevitable turn down the devil's path where ghosts and goblins are the real culprit of every problem. This is an instance where god becomes a convenient shield for us to hide behind and protect ourselves. Keep in mind that all stories that are told by anyone are filtered through whatever religious perspective the person holds. Remember--perspective is everything.

In any case, I recommended a few herbal supplements to help the brain's function and concentration to the mother with the ADD-symptomatic daughter. I had to tell her, yet again, how I felt and even offered to see her daughter for free at my office because of my genuine concern for her. The mother's excuse was that she lived too far away to come in for treatment and that she just needed something to get her daughter through school. In my office I would have used my own personal method of reaching deeper levels of energy blockages; greatly increasing the daughter' and the mother's ability to heal. I usually like to treat children with their parents because oftentimes, it is the parents who need to change more than the children.

When I know that someone's sickness is strongly emotionally based, it is difficult for me to just recommend an herbal band-aid just to get them out of my hair. This is where Naturopathy has gone wrong. There definitely is an herb for every sickness and symptom, but there is often a threshold that the herb meets within the human body. The herb on some level will be rejected or assimilated based on the organism's innate propensity to be healed. Put quite simply, does the organism really want to be healed?

A Case of Autism: My Son

Too often, the ever-changing information about Autism tries to cram the disease into a neat, predictable box. When I realized I had an autistic son (this was before he was actually diagnosed) I fought to prevent myself from believing it was true. My son was never vaccinated, I had nursed him for thirteen months and he ate a diet composed of organic foods. He would frequently hit his head with his fists, stare off into nothing, couldn't hear, couldn't talk, couldn't walk, and did not like to be touched. All of these symptoms seemed to come and go, appear together, or at other times, manifest separately. We took him from doctor to doctor and spent hundreds of thousands of dollars, running in circles.

One doctor that came highly recommended gave us a wrong diagnosis of hydrocephalus. Another doctor gave him a test to walk in a straight line and an MRI. We left the office with a diagnosis that our son was developmentally delayed. At that time we were searching for a diagnosis because we wanted to sue the obstetrician to get money for his treatments, which were costly. Ironically, the doctors were more than happy to diagnosis him after he reached the age of limitations, which means after a certain number of years you can no longer sue. We eventually found out that his skull was broken at birth from the vacuum extraction. He was suffering from bouts of excruciating pressure, migraine headaches from fascia around his skull that was squeezing and restricting his skull bones and nerves.

He had also suffered from chronic diarrhea since birth. This led us on another separate journey to try to heal his intestines. The most highly respected pediatric gastroenterologist in our state gave us the diagnosis that it was childhood diarrhea and he would simply "grow out of it". Following this, we had him tested for celiac disease two times.

During our medical excursions we were aggressively searching out every alternative treatment for our child I could find. Most alternative doctors blamed his symptoms and diarrhea on allergies. We got rid of our two dogs, changed all of our cleaning products, and the replaced the lights in our house. We spent thousands of dollars on vitamins and herbs from various "recommended naturopaths," most of who were chiropractors. Not one of them ever admitted to not knowing what was wrong with him when they finally then ended up referring us elsewhere. To the contrary, each one of these doctors was quite confident that they knew exactly what was wrong with him. We always left the offices excited but completely misled, not to mention $200 to $500 poorer and we rode this ferris wheel for a few years. This was until I got further on in my own studies and I was ready to open my eyes and deal with what was really going on.

We eventually found out that the chronic diarrhea was not caused by allergies as we had thought. The broken bones in his skull were putting pressure and damaging nerves leading from the head to the stomach. With a few osteopathic manipulations on his skull and intense craniosacral therapy, his chronic diarrhea cleared up, his speech dramatically improved, and he was able to start writing instead of scribbling. His ability to be present in the moment improved after I went through Orgonomy with him and effectively attached myself emotionally to him.

I can say with all confidence that it was the darkest hour for my family—that time when our child was alone in a world of pain and no one in the medical realm wanted to get involved for fear of blowing the whistle on a fellow doctor. All the doctors around us cared more about protecting each other in their blatant negligence then they cared about the life of an innocent child. I was very hurt, but the truth was that all of this had only further served to cement the feelings and suspicions I already carried about the medical realm. I tried to do everything and I felt I had protected my child from the dangers I knew existed within the standard medical propaganda concerning vaccination. This would only have left him wide open and vulnerable to be attacked by disease at his birth.

You might be wondering why I even had a hospital birth in the first place, especially given my concerns and realizations about standard medical practice. I will admit that the decision was against my better judgment at the time. I let fear overtake me and had not developed the trust and confidence that I have in my body now. Those learned attributes were taught to me through my journey into and through motherhood. Unfortunately, my son's birth will always be what I view as the biggest failure and biggest catalyst for change in my life. I spent years in a state of personal guilt and agony because of it, and so did my son. Interestingly, my son has a slew of friends the same age with similar problems, all of whom had different types of births. One of the friends had a C-section birth, had her child vaccinated, and he now has the same symptoms. There are many mysteries and since my battle, I have tried to get to the root of the causes and contributors to these similar symptoms.

Many people I know with autistic children are convinced that autism is caused by allergies and to combat this, they choose to keep their children on a strict diet. These children are often put on a severely restricted gluten/dairy-free diet. The gluten diet works by not agitating the body's immune response system. The diet, then, merely appeases and placates the disease. My friend's son goes right back into his autistic episodes whenever he goes off of his diet. Because of the conditions they have set for themselves, the boy and his family are literally prisoners in their home because of that restricted diet.

Allergies and Autism

I raise two questions about children who have allergy-induced autism. First of all, where do these allergies come from? To me, the answer is complex and is not just rooted in one cause or trigger. More specifically, vaccination has mutated our genetic structure. I base this on the simple fact that vaccines are mixed with the genetic material from the animal kingdom. In the case of the polio vaccine, it is mixed with monkey kidney and calf serum. The ever popular, MMR, contains chick embryo and biological materials from other animal cells (Miller, 1999). Apart from receiving different vaccines that have altered us biologically, we all have been raised with pesticides and poisons in our air and in our food. In short, we have been contaminated from within and from the outside world.

It is important to realize a few things about the ingredients and components of vaccines to best understand what it is we have been carrying in our bodies since we were children. Most vaccines are not only composed of harmful metals and carcinogens, but also the DNA of animals; chickens, and monkeys, etc. No one really understands or has studied the long-term effects on the human genetic structure when it is continually injected with animal DNA generation after generation. There is a link to these toxins that is passed on. I, a mother who was vaccinated and drugged constantly as a child, had a child who is directly affected by my life-long partnership with the pharmaceutical, food, petroleum and chemical industries.

The second question I ask regarding autism is this: what are these precious little souls coming into this world to teach us? After all, each soul comes in or came in with a cosmic purpose. Perhaps autistic children are trying to make society more aware of the choices we make (or don't make), how we raise our children, and how we either restrict or allow in the poisons we put into our body. It's as if the ADD generation in the eighties did not make a great enough impact, so now autism rears its ugly head. Many people have become aware of the terms "indigo children" or "crystal children." There are several books and even a movie called the "Indigo Children" available on the subject. The information is valuable if only to help parents realize how special their children are and to stop viewing them as societal rejects or problem children. One can look at the story of Helen Keller and see how easy it is to abuse these children who are not exactly like us out of frustration or parental guilt and shame.

What many people do not know is that research has shown that as many as 30% of children's autism can be alleviated by mothers actively [lovingly and sincerely] holding their children and making eye contact with them (Welch, 1988). This goes to show that at birth there can be insufficient bonding between the mother and child. In the book *Holding Time*, Dr. Martha Welch provides a simple holding technique that allows a mother to "re-bond" with her child. In this book she provides all of the research and information that will help mothers actively provide the emotional needs of their children. This book's "new" research directly coincides with and supports Reich's research from 70 years ago, so with all of this time-worn information, why then do we still ignore it? We ignore it because we want to believe that bad genes and the bad decisions of other people have made our children sick. We ignore it because we are in the habit of keeping ourselves as far away from our children's healing as possible.

The holding that Dr. Welch recommends is *inadequate* without the treatment of Orgonomy. The child must be able to scream and physically get the trauma out of the body by kicking and hitting a pillow or bed. If anything, "holding" opens the door to truth and contact between parent and child and yes, if the parent is angry or hostile toward the child or even feels those emotions, the holding will backfire. In short, what this means is that if you are angry and haven't worked through your own problems, your child will interpret what you are doing as cruel and not loving. On my end, I can tell you that personally, the only thing that worked was for me, the Mother, to actively engage in hitting and kicking my anger out before I held my child. Many times this allowed me to really contact my child in his eyes and even cry myself. Children are really much more forgiving than we give them credit for. They want to forgive and they wait for us to meet them—honestly.

I recognize that there are some people who are uncomfortable with holding their child and lack the confidence to reach out and face possible rejection—after all, I was one of them. I actually received an email recently, from a distraught mother of an autistic child proclaiming "holding your child is against the law!" Obviously, there is a lot of anxiety and false information in this area. For instance, there is controversy in the autistic realm about something called the "refrigerator mom syndrome" that comes from back in the early 1900s. This is when doctors were blaming mothers who were already overly taxed with large families with too many children, too many chores and not enough human rights for the autism of their children. RM syndrome has since been discredited. However, I logically do not discredit it due to the time period and circumstance. It does not seem strange to me that a mother of 8 or 12 children possibly married to a man she doesn't love, might reject one of her children or even a few of her children. While the RM syndrome label denotes a "bad" mother and should not be used. The fact that Dr. Welch's modern research still correlates with some of the aspects of the older theories should not be ignored either.

I also want to mention in defense Dr. Welch's work, that her holding therapy is nothing like some of the modern aggressive medical holding treatments which borderline abuse such as ABA and various others like it. These include forceful aggressive treatments by doctors and parents in which they hold children down, and sometimes even bind them. I want to make it clear that I am *not* referring to this at all. I cannot stress enough that I am an activist for the mother/child relationship and that healing the relationship between mother and child with love and empowered parenting is necessary. A parent that is willing to look at the child, cry, hug them and say "I don't care if you hate me, I am bigger and stronger than that, I LOVE YOU." This is a type of strength and maternal self-confidence that can help heal any illness, not just autism. All I can say now is that if the information I present upsets you and makes you angry, then please explore the possibility of getting help for your child's sake.

In Reich's book *Children of the Future* autism is described in context of children presenting with falling anxiety. Keep in mind that autism in the 1950s was strongly psychosomatic as children were not inundated with the host of toxic chemicals that surround the infant's environment today. Even still, the information he presents is just as relevant now as it ever was. According to Reich, it is the adults' lack of understanding of the newborns expressive language which causes the child to "go in" and withdraw, as in the case of autism and ADD. In other words, Reich describes autism as an artifact created by the behavior of the adults (Reich, 1967). A newborn's anxiety about falling also stems from the child picking up on the mother's anxiety and lack of confidence with her child.

Reich maintained that as long as parents, doctors, and educators approached infants with false, unbending behavior, inflexible opinions, condescension and officiousness, instead of with (real, genuine, loving, accepting) contact, infants will continue to be quiet, withdrawn, apathetic, autistic, peculiar, and later "little wild animals" with whom the adults feel that they have to "tame."

Essentially, Reich says that the world will not change, despite all of the political talk, as long as grownups fail to take the trouble to dissolve their own armors and defenses from influencing the spontaneous, free nature of the their children. Reich goes so far as to describe the reason causing the physical metabolic imbalances found in such diseases of autism and ADD. The deficiencies of inner secretions and inhibited enzyme functions, he said, are the direct results and symptoms--not the causes of--later diseases of the biosystem. He poignantly described social misery as being created by stiff and hardened human beings [emotionally deadened] that have no understanding of what is actually alive, in fact, they fear it.

On the topic of "social misery" Reich suggests that there is no kind of social misery to equal the misery of the infants with biopathic (armored) parents. He expounded by stating that in our world, there is always enough money for wars but never enough for our most important war--the protection of life. Reich was not talking about abortion protestors and subsidized government programs, he was talking about the investment and time spent between parents and children to truly bond with and accept their children; starting in utero and following through out their life. The basic needs of an infant all center on protection and include limiting harmful birthing practices, allowing the child to be born in a loving and natural environment, and nursing the child. Then, the even more simplistic needs of the children are to just touch, feel, and express how they feel. All of this is expected to come from a mother that is consciously aware of her body, birth, and her own issues that might block these experiences from being productive, healthy, and open. It seems to be painfully obvious that the simpler the needs of the infant and child are, the harder they are to be protected and given allowance for by the adults.

The book I mentioned earlier, *Saharasia* by Dr. James DeMeo, is a must-have for anyone with children or planning to have children. This epic took Dr. DeMeo ten years to research and write. In this text, he documents and provides timely information on the residual effects of cultural infant abuse-such as female and male genital mutilation and harmful parenting techniques that include ignoring infant cries, strict feeding schedules, shaming practices, and corporal punishment. DeMeo's book is a refreshing change in a culture that has become once again engaged in medieval ideas about contraception, childbirth, and raising children. It was upon reading that book that I was brought to tears and finally came to the difficult realization that I must take responsibility for my own personal contributions to my child's problems.

In the end, my child was healed of his autism through the use of a variety of therapies. Besides the intense osteopathic manipulations and craniosacral therapy for his skull, he also went through an aluminum detox because he had heavy metal poisoning. The most necessary therapy was by far Orgonomy. This therapy released the birth trauma rage and emotional scarring. Circumcision and a drugged traumatic birth were some of the issues he was clinging to deep within his body. When the pressure in his head from the broken bones was finally relieved, the emotional component became imperative. He had a deep resentment towards me and he didn't even know why. Through Orgonomy we were able to find out that he held me, his mother, responsible for his birth. He felt the deep pain of having his birthday stolen from him (induction), of being forcibly removed from his mother's womb (vacuum, drugs, forceps, c-section), of being held down under bright lights and poked and prodded like an inanimate voodoo doll, and the horror of being held down and being genitally mutilated. Orgonomy was important for me as well, so I could help him without getting caught up in my own deep shame and resentment towards myself.

The emotional component is often the hardest for mothers to look at and admit to or recognize. Many families would gladly spend thousand of dollars on herbs, special foods, and medications rather than address and take responsibility for their child's emotional needs. My son and I are now enjoying a true mother-child relationship and we are on the road to not just healing the body, but to healing the mind. Indeed, the hardest part of my son's autism did not begin and end with a broken bone in his head but was first and foremost begun with a broken heart. A mother who did not know or trust her own body and a child who was an innocent victim in the monopoly of birth, drugs, money and lies—these elements create a toxic situation but there are ways to recover, grow, and heal.

The Good News and the Bad

You may have noticed already that my style of writing is very "no holds barred" and I leave no stone unturned. It can be comforting because you will always know exactly where I stand but at the same time, it can be a jarring experience to read and face some of these issues head-on. The material presented here can serve as a type of "good news with the bad news" reading, depending on who encounters any particular section of the book.

With this in mind, after discussing the importance of a mother bonding with her child and reaching out to meet and know them, I must now mention the "other" side of this story--the mother that appears to be too bonded to her child. I urge you to consider that it may not be the case, despite appearances. While on the outside, this type of mother we speak of may look like she is a giving mother superior--nursing all day and sleeping with her children all night. You maybe thinking, can one be too close to their child?

The truth is, the matter of being "too close" depends on the individual parent and what the unconscious motives and intentions are. If the parent is indeed anxiety ridden, has something to prove, or refuses to let the child go then, yes, the closeness is not about love but again, about insecurity.

You may start to see that what we are talking about here are two sides of the same coin: the smothering mother that holds her child back and on the reverse side, the detached mother who cannot or will not connect. The lesson for all mothers is the word *temperance*. Of course, there is a time to sleep with your baby, nurse your baby, hold your baby but equally, there is also a critical time for the baby to grow and experience life. When the time comes for the baby to make the transition into childhood and then again into adulthood, the mother must be strong enough and confident enough to carry the child through to the next transition, supporting the child, guiding the child and leading the way.

There are many different motives behind why a mother will not help to transition her child through healthy life stages. In its most neurotic form you have an actual emotional incest where the mother is relying on the child emotionally--like a spouse or more. This is too much for a child to handle and will likely cause severe psychological damage in their adulthood.

In its most delicate form you have a mother who simply doesn't trust herself and is perhaps combating her own strict childhood through her child. In this way, the mother tries so hard to do opposite of what her parents did that eventually, it comes full circle and has a truly disastrous effect. Because of the lack of boundaries and rhythm in these households the children grow up feeling very insecure, having missed some important rites of passage in childhood.

Recreating Tribal Cultures

Many child-centered parents will use the excuse of trying to live and recreate an ancient tribal culture for their children. This idea sounds idyllic; sharing a family bed and nursing the child until the age of six--but this concept has been researched and, for the most part, disproven. One such source that provides insight about why this tribal form of parenting is not viable can found in the work of Jean Liedloff, who is a pioneer of the modern movement for western women to nurse and wear their babies. She based her ideas on the child-rearing philosophies of the Yequana Indians, whom she lived with and derived her research from. Her article about the Mother/child relationship in modern culture is a tribute to her ability to promote a balanced perspective in motherhood. Liedloff did what many other researchers would not do; she went back during a series of revisions and disproved parts of her information and discussed in detail how and why it wasn't working and how it could be improved.

Her re-discovery was that extended nursing/baby-wearing by western mothers and related child-centered practices were not working. The women had become so polarized and imbalanced that the children were turning selfish (and as she termed) "demanding brats." This idea bears direct similarities to the deaf and blind woman, Helen Keller--her mother's continual giving in to her made her resent her mother. It actually stopped Helen's learning and kept her from progressing to higher levels of maturity

Liedloff's article, "Who's in Control" explores the idea of creating children many could term "spoiled" by stating, "It appears that many parents of toddlers, in their anxiety to be neither negligent nor disrespectful, have gone overboard in what may seem to be the other direction"(Liedloff, 1994). We are at clearly at historical crossroads; where east meets west and where the Victorian era meets the industrial, technological new Age of Aquarius. If nothing else is clear, it is that a new way forward is necessary.

The research by Jean Liedloff and the story of Helen Keller spans across all lines of race, class and religion. It is not isolated solely within the topic of nursing and child-wearing, but is present in all areas of our life, particularly within the fields of health and education. It is our imbalanced lifestyle that keeps us from being better mothers and keeps us from living the healthy life that we deserve.

Chapter 3

Naturopathy: Where it's Going, Where it's Gone...

Natural health has become established as a trend in our society, especially in the last decade. These days, it seems as if almost every label has the word "natural" on it and is packaged and marketed using the most innocuous language about purity and health. However, if you read these labels you will often find a list of undesirable ingredients—they are those ones that you cannot pronounce. Most of these ingredients are toxic to our health and well-being and any product that claims to be natural yet still contains complex words that designated chemical compounds is anything but directly from the earth.

The actor Tom Cruise made national headlines when he declared that anti-depressants are not necessary or natural for anyone. On the one hand, he might be right--if we only addressing how people are consciously aware of their bodies and feelings to such a degree that they have no need for those anti-depressants or any other kind of drug. But the truth is, in our world, that awareness is not particularly present. After childbirth, for example, a few can enter a postpartum depression so severe that they actually want to kill the children to whom they have just given birth. This is not a symptom we can ignore by wishing it away; it is a serious problem. Currently, our course of action is to offer drugs. In our world, we choose drugs almost every time. It is what we know or think will work. We have been conditioned to trust the "un-trustable."

Tom Cruises allegations about anti-depressants were shrugged off as a bizarre, inconceivable announcement, but were they really? In May 2000, The *New Yorker* posted a startling article called the "Empty Couch" about the detriment of drug use in psychiatry. This not only backs up what Tom Cruise stated, but supported the belief with research and hard facts that drugs are not the best and only choice. The *New Yorker* article is based on two books, "Of Two Minds: The Growing Disorder in American Psychiatry" by T. M Luhrmann and a book by a Harvard medical school psychiatrist, Joseph Glenmullen, entitled "Prozac Backlash."

By combining research by such highly credible sources, the article successfully chronicles the horrors and atrocities of modern psychiatric medicine and suggests that people are conveniently sedated and never truly healed or released from their psychological disorders. Furthermore, it details the devastating long-term and short-term side effects from using psychiatric drugs. One of the serious side-effects listed was the presence of swollen thick and severely malformed brain cells in rats after they had been on the drugs Prozac or Zoloft for only four days (Acocella, 2000). Four days!

Speaking of alternative methods, there is another way to address symptoms of severe depression and other illnesses without drugs. This method is one in which we seek to find out what it is that underlies the problem in the first place, and in so doing, help people discover avenues by which they can learn how to heal themselves. This concept which I term "naturopathic psychotherapy" is explored more definitively in the final chapter. Drugs have caused many in our society to sleep through life and reality, and we are accustomed to using them from the moment of birth. People in this country believe they need the medications given to them by the medical profession and without more developed information, do not acknowledge that other alternatives exist. The vast majority of people are not willing to delve deeper into the root causes of their problems or to look at the ingredients in the drugs they are feeding their systems. What would happen to our children or to the entire country, for that matter, if everyone stopped taking their medications? Sedation through drugs keeps society moving along in a sort of numbingly predictable, lethargic flow. So, yes we still need drugs—at least until we are ready to fully come into and integrate into our life and reality.

Another process that Tom Cruise insisted was important was having a silent birth. He seemed to be genuinely concerned about the importance of bringing children into the world with conscious awareness throughout gestation and labor. Despite the fresh round of criticism that was heaped upon him after making such an unorthodox suggestion, to me, conscious birth is important and makes perfect sense. What does not make sense, however, is that all of the various efforts to ensure the peaceful birth with no "sound" was rendered meaningless when he continually advocated the use of ultrasound and doppler on the fetus in-utero. I have long been against the use and overuse of ultrasound in pregnancy for many reasons. I have read compelling research that ultrasound causes cell mutation (Doida, Brayman, and Miller, 1992) and most recently that ultrasound contributes significantly to autism, delayed speech and birth defects of the genitals (Rogers, 2006). These studies are not widely known or publicized, as they are not sponsored by the multi-million dollar ultrasound business. In 1993 however, The Canadian Medical Association Journal, The Lancet, and the New England Journal of Medicine brought the dangers of ultrasound into question (Wagner, 1999).

Within the American public's reach is finally a study produced by a highly respected physician of the Mayo Clinic, Dr. Mostafa Fatemi. To preface this discussion, I should mention that I came across Dr. Fatemi's research in the most unusual way. Several news channels ran stories about babies "moving" during ultrasound. They described Doctor Fatemi's research as showing that babies move a little from the "slight vibrations" that the ultrasound creates. Gently describing the sound as rain drops on an umbrella (Wu, 2002).

Just reading these news articles made alarm bells go off in my head regarding the fetus and water. I remembered being scolded as a child for tapping on fishing aquariums. The reason given was because the barely-audible tap resonated and amplified in the water. Tapping on the aquarium would scare the fish and damage the fishes' hearing. Upon considering this, I remembered how last year my three-year-old son was scolded at a pet store for tapping on a plastic aquarium full of feeder goldfish. My first response after reading these articles was, "Wow, so much concern over sound waves and fish, but little or no concern for human embryos." I decided to do some more research.

I easily found doctor Fatemi's research, which was available through the Mayo Clinic's website. The article was much more disturbing then the media had led on in those pieces in the news. For example, Alan Neis, an ultrasound technician describes fetal ultrasound as high-frequency sound waves that operate at about 100 decibels!? That might not carry a full impact for you if you consider it in detached decibel levels, so let me make a comparison. For us, 100 decibels is the equivalent of a chain saw, a rock concert, and as Dr. Fatemi reports, a train coming at you at close range. To arrive at his conclusions, Dr. Fatemi measured the sound levels within the womb (Fatemi, 2006). One of the articles that rehashed these findings went on to say, that doctors have witnessed babies trying to reach up and cover their ears when ultrasound was applied (Williams, 2006). We have, yet again, another example, of how our health and access to information has been manipulated by corporations, medicine and the media.

Abortion: The Truth and Nothing But the Truth

On the subject of harmful fetal practices, we also need to address the controversial topic of abortion. We may all agree that abortion is unfortunate and wrong in ways that are all-encompassing or in situational terms, depending on our individual perspectives. However, it seems clear that abortion is not a simple black or white issue. In fact, the root causes of abortion lie in basing our future on truthful and honest education, not in limiting or stopping the ability of women to get the procedure. An important key to the abortion dilemma is early detection and early termination.

Unwanted pregnancies happen; this is a fact of life and it is difficult to understand why more people are not being honest about that reality. In a perfect society, or at least in an enlightened one, women will know how their bodies function inside and out. They will be taught about fertility and menstruation at an early age by their mothers and grandmothers. They will be initiated into womanhood not from a perspective emphasizing fear and shame, but one that passes on a sense of pride and joy. From this premise, women will be able to raise their sons to honor fertility and women's bodies and not use and abuse them. Unwanted pregnancies will then become the exception, not the norm.

Coincidently, beyond the subject of abortion, it is significant that few people raise an eyebrow at the reality of married women in the U.S. who will continue to have unwanted children out of guilt or because they adhere to a religious dogma. Surely, that is just as relevant an issue as abortion. While we may challenge abortion because it ends life, surely we should also be challenging the readiness with which we allow children to be born to mothers who do not want them. This is a reality for many women—and one that causes immense trauma to the child throughout the entire course of life. Hence, the issue of unwanted children should be a topic of discussion as much as abortion itself. My book "Waking the American Dream" delves deeply into the aspects of the mother/child connection and how it affects health.

Man Against the Machine

Teaching and guiding others into knowing and accepting their bodies is the ancient Naturopathic way. Naturopathy has moved away from its ancient roots and is beginning to compete with standard medicine, albeit in strangely familiar ways. For instance, many naturopaths now rely heavily on electronic gadgets and computers, seeking to impress their patients through this process that clearly seeks to legitimize their practice, at least in the eyes of their patients. Some naturopaths are becoming dependent on the machine to do what they no longer want to do. When all is said and done, naturopathy has not evolved as much as it simply melded into the framework of the medical millennial machine. While many electronic devices can prove useful, any good naturopath doctor can effectively understand the patient's condition and how to treat it within a few minutes without the use or need for any mechanical devices. For naturopathy, the goal should never be to diagnose and solidify our horror and disbelief in the power of healing the human body. The goal always needs to be directed and devoted to a creating a balance to help individuals work toward health.

Ayurveda is one alternative path for accomplishing a rapid assessment of the patient's condition. I use pulse diagnosis to find imbalances, which is an ayurvedic technique. I use what is termed a "symptom inventory" to reconfirm my diagnosis. Using this process, I can know how to treat a condition and restore a balance in the body within a matter of minutes. The only problem with this is that many people are conditioned to only trust the machine. It is what they are accustomed to seeing used; they want and need to know about their sickness on a screen in big letters. I was taught in naturopathy never to focus on diagnosing the disease but rather, to focus on balancing the body. I have to stand by that precept and work with my patients by teaching and guiding them to trust innately in themselves. True healing comes through and within them, not through or from me.

My Own Experience with a Naturopath

Before I got seriously involved in my studies and Ayurveda, I visited a Naturopathic consultant. I wanted to get a reading on one of the new diagnostic machines that had become available to diagnose illness (which is actually against the law in the States for Naturopaths). I had lost a fingernail as a result of one of my recurring candida infections and this was what originally prompted me to make an appointment. At first, I searched through the area phone book, but to no avail, thus my search had to continue online. That gave me a few leads, but I felt unsure about the information I retrieved, so after my other options had been exhausted, I just decided to rely solely on word-of-mouth.

When I finally found someone via recommendations, the woman I spoke to first seemed genuinely concerned about my condition .She was also kind enough to move some appointments around to get me in right away.

She practiced out of her home, which was more than sixty miles from mine. My husband came home from work early so that he could watch our three children. I set out around noontime and arrived at her residence a little after 1:30 pm. This was after taking some wrong turns and calling for directions a few times on my cell phone. Over the phone, her husband graciously led me through subdivision after subdivision. He greeted me at the front door and led me to her office. She was a small 70-year old woman, sitting at her desk. We shook hands and started our consultation.

The first thing she had me do was leave a urine and saliva sample in the bathroom so she could test my pH. Afterwards, I sat down in her office to fill out four pages of paperwork and history. One sheet was specifically for thyroid disorders, the other specifically for candida, and the other two for lifestyle, diet, and major health concerns. She then hooked me up to a machine called Maitreya that was programmed into her computer. This procedure is similar to biofeedback--straps were placed around my head, arms, and ankles to obtain the readings.

I remember that I was definitely surprised at the level of accuracy the machine reading produced. It appeared to be reading my mind and every organ of my body. The machine knew that I had chicken pox six months prior and pneumonia three weeks before. It also showed the last time I drank water and that my neck would "go out" in two days (it really did!). She spent about a half-hour going through different organs with me on the computer. She zoomed in and showed me that I had a low thyroid disorder and how what percentage of my ailment was from toxins, radiation, miasms, and viral damage. She then used Maitreya to show the electromagnetic field around my body. She pulled up a list of my top ten worst allergens. The machine even showed the overall emotional problem that was causing my health problems. While all of this is certainly amazing, I feel I should mention that the machine itself produces its own damaging electromagnetic field as well.

This naturopathic doctor spent some time showing me that my sugar level was too high and that I needed to go off all sugar. For this she recommended a very expensive dietary drink. She also told me my urine was too acid and my saliva was too alkaline. To remedy this, she proposed that I take very expensive enzymes with each meal. On top of my severe candida infection, I also had parasites, hyperglycemia, and a hypothyroid. She made a chart of dietary recommendations to help me recover from these issues. In her basement she had an amazing array of excellent homeopathic remedies from all over the world and she carried the finest brands of herbal supplements and vitamins. All of this information proved invaluable to me, until the very end. Because it wasn't until the end that I felt the consultation went wrong.

The end of our session proved to be demoralizing as with the information she gained, I got the impression that she was using my symptoms as an opportunity to proselytize. She told me I needed to see the movie "The Passion" and recommended that I go to church. It was an incredible turn of events and I felt that I had been thrown completely off the course I was expecting to take.

I was offended that she judged my level of spirituality without even knowing me. Clearly, she assumed I was a depraved sinner. I couldn't help but wonder how the machine was somehow programmed to meet a fundamentalist perspective. Our conversation came to a head when her husband came into the room and interrupted us with a racist remark about the neighbors. This further discredited her evangelization process and greatly ruined any progress I felt we made to that time in the consultation. The only point she could have effectively made to me by then was that she did not love or accept anyone.

So that was how it went--I had just spent $500 to allow someone to make me feel worse than before I came in. In no way during our three hours did I ever feel loved or personally cared for by this woman. I also never received the impression that this woman was, in fact, a healer of any kind—she was simply a businesswoman with an evangelical mission. What this naturopath had was a "niche" within the naturopathic realm; she had learned how to effectively use this Maitreya machine and master a few kinesiology techniques—but this was a basic amount of training, just enough, in fact, to allow her to fulfill her broader objectives. Her broad spectrum knowledge about nutrition was applied to everyone and was not individually based. She used people's illness to create another "notch in her belt for her religion" rather than leading her clients towards freedom and health.

    I learned quite a bit from my visit to this particular naturopathic consultant. I definitely believe that to be an effective naturopath you have to simultaneously be a healer—it is only by having feet in both worlds that you can be effective. On my part, I can say that I consider myself to be a healer. The term healer, at least according to my own definition, denotes the ability to step out of one's own ego box and remove all judgment. Upon stepping out of this box, one can reach out and touch the life of another human being. I believe this is an essential step in any and all healing processes. This is the bridge between client and consultant. Acceptance, eye contact and touch will build the trust that is necessary to initiate the healing process. If sick individuals are threatened and judged by the very people that they come to for help, they can be left feeling alone, abandoned, and even more isolated in their illness than they were before. After all, these factors are often the very reason they are sick in the first place.

    I extend healing love to everyone in my personal practice as a naturopathic consultant. What does that mean? It means to put it quite simply, offering unconditional acceptance. Loving people and accepting people as they are is extremely healing in and of it's self. When we harshly judge individuals who walk into our office, a high, solid wall is instantly created and the session is essentially wasted before it's even begun. In order to effectively guide a nation of sick individuals back into health, we must not make gross, biased, and personal assumptions. This is where I believe the term "namaste" from yoga becomes all important. It means "the light in me bows to the light in you." The truth is that we all are filled with the light. This is without regard to race and religion. All of us deserve to be healthy.

This view may seem over-simplified but it deserves being stated. This issue of universal acceptance most certainly pertains to humanity's ability to heal itself at the present time--right now. A naturopathic consultant needs to have more than just a computer and a basement full of herbs. That person needs to have a heart.

The Thick and Thin of Naturopathy

As naturopaths, it is critical that we search ourselves, heal ourselves, and consciously look at ourselves without the self-deception that seems so inherent to our being whenever possible. In essence, we cannot help anyone unless we can help ourselves. Many people may find that premise narcissistic, but most assuredly it is not. Every person we come in contact with is directly affected by us, the naturopaths, and *not* by the herbs. Herbs are secondary to the healing and treatment patients receive at an office. Whether those patients go home, take their herbs, and follow the recommendations has a lot to do with the experience they have in that office.

When we reach out to help others, the love and healing desire we have goes through a huge "plastic" funnel. It is siphoned out through a tiny hole and somehow has to trickle its way to the opening in the heart and mind of the client/patient. The more aware that naturopaths are of their own limits, including those related to personality characteristics and health conflicts, the more capable they are of truly helping their patients and truly, changing the world.

Healing the Chronic Naturopathically

One reason that healing the chronically ill still eludes the natural health community is not just because of their generalized focus on competing with medical machines I've discussed. It is also because of the large scale avoidance of true naturopathic foundations in favor of easier symptomatic treatments which virtually ignore the core issues. In Orgonomy and Homeopathy there is a common belief that, on a strictly emotional level, allergy and chronic disease share similar psychosomatic cores. For instance, this is at the heart of the issue when there is extreme sensitivity, such as in the case of chronic disease and the type of overarching allergic reaction in which everything on the outside of the human becomes an "irritant." The body is following the mind in blocking itself and/or "reacting" violently to the outside world.

One of the founders of homeopathy, Hahnemann, conducted research of the Psora, which is the allergic miasm and is related to these overwhelming allergies to "life" itself. Different branches on the psora miasm tree are that the person will block themselves in the sinuses (mezereum) or in the throat (lachesis, argentum nitricum). This is the psychosomatic aspect of chronic illness and is in no way representative of a full and complete picture but is applicable nonetheless. The other aspect of allergy and chronic disease is one of habitual suppression of constitutional and or acute inflammatory responses as explained by a medical doctor, Dr. Henry Lindlahr in his book "Natural Therapeutics." It is an important work on natural health that was written over 100 years ago. I was taught this amazing information in school and as much as I believe it, live it and have witnessed it, it still completely escapes me why modern naturopaths ignore this information as a whole.

The Body is Forced *Not to* Heal

While Lindlahr's work and research is fairly "old," like Reich, the answers he provided to truly heal the core of illness have never fully been embraced. Lindlahr stood for the belief in the power of the human immune system to heal itself. Although this may initially sound like a Christian Scientist point of view, he differed from them by taking a firm stance on being proactive with health and maintaining the body's healing capacities. Because his ideas and research encouraged the important step of personal responsibility at a time when the dream of chemical medicine concoctions were the hope of tomorrow, much of it has lied dormant. Below I will briefly discuss his stance on chronic illness and compare it to mine so you can see the delicate blend of pertinent ideas that have comprised a philosophy that I know works—and I know *how* works. I stand by this information because I have tested it myself and used it for many years.

The allergy and chronic disorder can be likened to the body "turning on the switch" but there is a "short in the wire or a blown fuse from the panel." This ineffective, continual attempt of the body to throw off disease in allergic response is caused by the suppression of childhood fever. If the body was allowed in childhood to burn off disease from within (constitution) and without (epidemic predisposition) through effective and complete inflammatory response which is the fever; chronic illness, in the form of allergies, ear infection, systemic candida and rash would be obsolete or at least not so commonly prevalent. Notice if you will, the common way the human body expresses allergic reaction—it is almost indistinguishable from a cold except there is no acute fever. Although I am a strong advocate against inoculation, the first treatment given after vaccine, even if no symptoms are presented, is Tylenol or ibuprofen to suppress fever. Remembering my days as a pediatric nurse, I would give a vaccine and also dispense children's Tylenol immediately afterward in the office then I would also give the parent a "free" sample to dispense to the children at home as well. This was done in an effort to reduce the possibility of a vaccine reaction, thus effectively protecting the doctor that I worked for from being held responsible, pulled into a court room, or simply reporting reactions to the CDC. Talk about taking matters into my own hands…

To Help or To Hurt?

Ironically, in American inoculation, disease is introduced into the system (along with carcinogens along with animal and human DNA) then the efforts that the body makes to burn off the disease and chemically break it down is also completely blocked. Even if mass inoculation could theoretically work, the means by which the medical community uses to protect itself with the overuse and prescription of NSAIDs for necessary childhood illness compromises its entire foundation. This foundation was built on the idea or "medical legend" that the human body is too weak and stupid to heal itself. This idea, which is offensive to the entire human race, is slowly becoming a depressing fact in humanity's present degenerated and chronic state. Was this medical legend an allopathic prophecy or a seed that has been planted and is now slowly evolved and grown generation after generation? I propose this seed was planted within the minds and bodies of the last several generations. It has contributed to the emergence of new diseases where the immune system, not only fails to work, but actually attacks itself as in the case of lupus, rheumatoid arthritis, AIDS, and other auto-immune disorders.

Healing the Chronic

In my own work as a naturopath, I have successfully healed chronic disease only when there was an effective inflammatory response during treatment. The inflammatory response time follows the expression of inflammation during the sixth week of treatment during which I had subsequently employed dietary changes, color, herbs, homeopathy, and emotional release. It has been my experience that unless the person is committed to "healing the chronic" and following the previously mentioned treatments then results are still beneficial but will remain limited. When I read that Dr. Lindlahr saw the sixth week of an inflammatory response as a turning point in chronic illness, I never thought that healing could be so black and white. Yet, no matter what means are employed to heal chronic issues, my own experience has also proven what Lindlahr proved over 100 years ago--that inflammation is a friend of the body and is a necessary means to healing.

The Cause of Disease

The cause of disease in naturopathic philosophy can be explained by dividing disease into two groups: the acute and the chronic. Dr. Henry Lindlahr's book states that both acute and chronic disease have "bacteria" in common, however, it is the individual's "fertile soil" which allows bacteria to proliferate and disease and poisons to accumulate.

If this is the case, then what makes for fertile soil? It is the debilitating and empty diet of the western populace that has plagued generation after generation and continually gets worse. 100 years ago, in Dr. Lindlahr's time, diet was a major aspect of disease as it was considered a technological advance to boil milk, buy flour already milled, and eat large amounts of meat with cooked vegetables. These actions saved time, but in the process destroyed enzymes, vitamins, and the life-giving energy of the food itself. All of the so-called dietetic advances of that time gave way to debilitating diseases of our great grandparents, dental carries, and laid "fertile soil" for a host of chronic problems for future generations.

A Modern Catastrophe

Moving forward into the later half of the 20th century, the same diet exists and is now considered "normal" and acceptable, even by the more naturopathically and healthy inclined. The 20th-century diet has added some of the most lethal and DNA-damaging poisons into the equation such as; food coloring, food preservatives, large amounts of depleted white sugar, flour and salt, non-hydrogenated oils, and the hormone-scrambling grain nouveau, the soybean. It is also important to mention the time bombs of irradiation, genetic modification, and pesticidation, all of which are dangerous trends in agricultural proliferation.

When considering the modern human as being both a fertile soil for disease and an infertile soil for health, one must keep in mind the additional immediate and long-term effects of the environment. The macrocosm of the universe effects the microcosm of the human organism. Outdoor pollution such as radiation from nuclear reactors and indoor pollution in the form of plastics, fluorescent bulbs and "cleaning" products are new disease-causers that were not even available in the already sick and malnourished man of the early 1900s.

Some products that directly affect the health and well-being of Americans have already been banned in other parts of the world. They are, as I have previously mentioned, fluorescent bulbs, certain brands of fabric protectors, flame retardants (notoriously sprayed on children's pajamas and furniture), water fluoridation, and of course, the many pesticides that are used on a wide variety of foods.

Most recently, it was scientifically proven that pesticides depleted a large amount of the American bee populations causing a 2006 mass colony collapse (Scott, 2009). To this the government scientists tell us, not to worry, it still cannot affect the humans.

The Auto-Immune Society

And so, with this information, we lay the backdrop for the acute and chronic--the modern millennially evolved auto-immune disorder. The question now becomes more complex as we ask questions about why so many acute diseases eventually give way to chronic illnesses. The answer lies within the simplicity of the inflammatory response. Dr. Henry Lindlahr stated that acute disease is the result of the purifying efforts of nature and that it runs its course based on the five stages of inflammation (Lindlahr, 1985). The five stages of inflammation are incubation, aggravation, destruction, abatement, and reconstruction. Because of modern day's reliance of anti-inflammatories such as NSAIDs, vaccines, antiseptics and antibiotics to inhibit and/or control the immune response, many acute conditions have become chronic.

Chronic disease is manifested through debilitated and weakened organs and genetic constitution. It is much harder to heal the acute, which is the sole reason why it is so urgent for modern man to change his immuno-suppressive ways. The constant thwarting of the natural and necessary healing response in the human body has affected the population and has partially, if not completely, already suppressed immune function over the course of generations.

Allopathic medicine has placated the chronically-ill masses by providing what can best be equated to a wolf in sheep's clothing; the immediate aesthetic benefits of health via suppressing fever, chasing germs, and identifying symptoms for a comfortable and easy "appearance" of health. However, the long-term harmful chronic effects far outweigh the immediate benefits of "fake" health. One can only look to a family member or neighbor to see the modern plagues of our time such as diabetes, MS, lupus, cancer, not to mention the constitutionally weakened new generation of children who are afflicted, to a large degree, by poor dentition (cavities), poor eyesight, and persistent ear infections. In addition to this host of conditions, chronic childhood disorders such as autism and arthritis are more prevalent everyday.

What does all of this mean? To begin with, we as members of an adult society, are clearly too comfortable with disease. We see it as something to be anticipated throughout the course of life and expected to happen to all of us at some point. But is that belief good and beneficial for our children and for the future of mankind?

Naturopathy Works.....

Naturopathic living works because it unifies the body and mind by bringing man back to nature and back to its core. It guides people towards healthy living by teaching others what they already know, what comes natural to them. By honoring the human body simple and effective natural means the person is empowered to heal themselves and treat illness not as a faceless monster but as a catalyst to a stronger and more fulfilling existence. Besides the long term disease preventative benefits, it also positively effects the future by blessing our offspring with knowledge and wisdom and not fear and disability. In this way, one can support the human body and mind by finally believing in its power rather than constantly trying to disprove it.

The story of the Pottinger cat experiment in Appendix VI of Lindlahr's book shows that it takes only a few generations of unhealthy living and eating to weaken an organism but many generations to build it back up to thriving sufficiency. Furthermore, the food experiment where animals fed white flour and white sugar died sooner than animals fed nothing was to me, shocking and sobering. However, this should not discourage us but inspire us to the urgency and dire need to lead a healthier life and make better choices for us and our families.

Chapter 4

Ancient Healing Meets New Disease

During my training, I found myself searching for the most economical healing methods. The practice of yoga, specifically the flowing movements and poses (asanas) of hatha, can be helpful on many different levels. Yoga is an ancient health program from India. It is an umbrella term that indicates many different practices daily life practices to heal the body and develop the mind. Despite many efforts to classify it religiously, it is not a religion but a series of comprehensive mental and physical practices. The word yoga in Sanskrit means oneness, thus revealing the ultimate goal of practicing it. It is a tangible practical system to develop the human in a conscious, harmonic and natural way (Janakananda, 1991).

I mention the term hatha yoga, which is a gentle, releasing breath flowing form of yoga because of the context of this book. The essence of yoga continues to become habitually disregarded and even lost to a great extent in the West. The flowing breaths and movements of hatha moves energy and feeling through the body. However, the rigid movements of modern yoga which can be described as mechanical, competitive and even painful shows that it has taking a divisive turn away from oneness. Aggressively holding poses and disruptively disassociating the breath from the body to increase strength and yogic "prowess" is a modern yoga travesty. My own form of bio-therapeutic yoga, which I mention later, is based on both hatha yoga and Orgonomy. Its goal is in keeping both in keeping with ancient precepts of yoga and our modern necessity of freeing up the humans rigid external and internal core.

I believe that in order to get the most out of yogic practice there has to be, at least initially, a form of emotional release and healing. Yoga and meditation can facilitate a release through body movements and awareness on their own to some extent. However, sat nam, which is a part of a yogic mantra (verbal affirmation) for personal truth, needs to be actively realized and applied. The basis for anything we do needs to be truth and honesty. Being honest and unashamed about our feelings and who we are is the most important aspect of healing. Yes, we can lie to people about who we are and how we feel, but never should we lie to ourselves. We need to work, constantly and earnestly, to become more self-aware and honest about ourselves to ourselves. For instance, I have seen yogic practitioners beat themselves up for feeling angry or upset. They view those emotions as a failure in their practice of yoga or as a block to enlightenment. As long as we recognize the self and what it needs, then yoga and meditation can be successfully implemented.

Is the process of hiding feelings, suppressing them, and actively pretending and lying about them meant to be a part of yoga practice? Swami Janakananda indicates in his book "Yoga" that suppressing human emotion in yoga was picked up recently by Victorian era thought which still purveys much of Western thinking. He also implies that many modern books on yoga mirror a fear of confronting life rather than accepting, experiencing, and actively participating in it (Janakananda, 1991).

Some other cost-effective modes of healing include magnets (used individually for less then two hours instead of inside a mattress, which is the current trend) sound, color, touch and aromatherapy. The sense of taste is enhanced by the use of the herbs and spices. I believe that it is most beneficial during any treatment to activate each one of the senses and each of these therapies do engage the five senses.

Touch is one of the more elusive, but intensely powerful senses. What should set any doctor or healer apart from another is the mode of "touch" he or she uses in treatment. Unfortunately, touching has been almost completely lost within our society. Many people are afraid to touch (again see Saharasia for information on mothers afraid to touch their own children). Illnesses and disease can respond positively from touch alone, one human being reaching out to another, in a sincere, non-mechanical way. Touch can be used in massage, craniosacral therapy, or even as just a gentle, reassuring squeeze on the arm.

Another interesting therapy that has emerged and has proven, at least in my experiences, to have some astonishing results is color therapy. Anyone can apply simple color techniques using what is called a "color light", which consists of nothing more than a few party lights and a goose-necked lamp. When I first found out about this mode of healing I was naturally quite skeptical until I saw it used to treat a friend of mine who was in excruciating pain with a toothache. The healer stopped the pain by using a piece of blue cellophane paper, which he wrapped around a flashlight before shining it on my friend's cheek. Later, I adopted the method and tested it on a sore throat: I used the color blue for an hour and to my surprise, my sore throat miraculously disappeared.

Since then, I too have been using color therapy in my practice and have found it to be extremely effective to treat a wide range of symptoms and ailments. I now use a more elaborate form of color therapy, treating the body with more than one color at a time with a machine I designed called the "Aurorachrome." With this machine I now have at my disposal a complete system of 7 different lights for the body and over 200 different color filter combinations. It is necessary for me to use a more elaborate device as I usually have two hours with each client during weekly visits. I have cut down the time it takes to heal considerably by using it. This is especially important when treating chronic disease which can take longer to heal than acute.

However, instead of withholding my knowledge, I teach my clients about the benefits of using color therapy at home and encourage them to make a small investment, from $20 to $100, so they can make it use of the techniques themselves, thus giving them ultimate control over their own healing at home.

Due to its ease of use and minimal investment, color therapy has been hijacked by scammers, schemers, and manipulators. All over the internet there are advertisements for expensive "color" machines for as much as $20,000! And why do you think these people charge so much? Simply because it works. Unfortunately, as with so many other previously inexpensive healing techniques and therapies, some people exploit it and sully its reputation.

Some people may find that these implements and techniques outlandish and too good to be true. Let me assure you that these gentle approaches are simply in tune with our bodies to begin with—light, magnets, and other natural healing tools are a part of our human physiology, not removed from it. If it seems overly simplified, well, quite honestly, it is. Since true healing comes from the mind first, it is only fitting that many of these practical therapies provide a catalyst that our bodies and minds need to reach and sustain balance. Million-dollar laboratory chemicals attempt to recreate synthetically what nature has already provided and perfected. This is because of the constant monopoly of healthcare, even within the naturopathic realm. We have come to believe that sickness should be expected and that good health comes with an expensive, inevitable price tag. The truth is that some of the most effective means to healing are also the cheapest.

Lights, Color, Sound, Action

Color therapy is probably the most economical, highly effective, and yet widely ignored treatment of our day. Though it can be utilized in many different ways one thing is certain, color physically and mentally affects the human body. The Waldorf school movement created by Rudolf Steiner uses color therapy based on the research of 18th century German scientist Goethe's work. The Ancient Indian vedic scriptures, in terms of Ayurveda, uses color therapy to balance the doshas, which are the elemental constitutions of the body: fire, water, or air.

More recently, another scientific application for color therapy was developed in the early 1900s. It is the work of the late Dr. Dinshah and his area of expertise "Spectro-chrome." Dinshah is attributed to bringing color therapy to the United States. He used color for healing many different diseases and also created a large case study database. Though he successfully worked and treated patients with spectro-chrome color therapy in a Philadelphia hospital, he was never free from persecution by the medical association who were out to prove he was a quack (Dinshah, 2005).

In my office, I use color therapy based on my extensive knowledge and research of Ayurveda, TCM (traditional Chinese medicine), Orgonomy and Spectro-chrome color therapy. The results are profound, relatively quick and no less than amazing. So much so, that I depend very little on expensive herbs and natural pills to bring the body back into balance. I have found, that though

Dinshah's protocol works effectively, it is also quite time consuming. The Aurorachrome machine, along with utilizing the schools of thought above, has allowed me to cut the result time considerably and even more favorably.

Dinshah referred to a color treatment session as a tonation, he also concluded with his research that the body or more specifically, the energetic shell surrounding the body, only takes the amount of color that it needs to balance. The body stops taking in color after an hour unless there is an acute problem, as in the case of hemorrhaging or sepsis (Dinshah, 2005). This is just one of the many foundational details of using Spectro-chrome color therapy

In Vedic or Goethe color therapy, problems arise when too much of one color upsets the balance on an emotional/energetic level (Thirta, 1998). For such devices as color-graded sunglasses, where you are continually receiving color, the mood or emotional body can become affected and altered. Take for example, pink glasses which have been used to reduce headaches and calm a person down within minutes. Bubblegum pink rooms are used in institutions and asylums in order to sedate and calm. One must also take into account the propensity for pink to continually relax or take an effect on someone who is too calm or lacking energy. Perhaps this could inadvertently contribute to apathy or the organism's ability to "enter in" to their life more consciously. In this way, grey gradient sunglasses are the best choice for daily use and any other colors should be reserved for special times and circumstances.

It's all about Waves

Like sound, color is a frequency or wave and can be measured. When comparing wave lengths, color has a much higher frequency than sound and for this reason it produces faster results. This wave phenomenon affects us on emotional and physical levels alike. For instance, in a bedroom lacking marital "action" it might very well be the color of the room or perhaps the bed is placed up against a wall inundated with electrical cords within the wall. Similarly, a TV, smoke detector, alarm clock, or computer could also be contributing to wavelength disorders, manifesting in a "bad" nights sleep or even in ways as complex as cancer and disease.

The scientific study of wavelengths is called cymatics. Under the umbrella term of cymatics there are both beneficial wavelengths and detrimental wavelengths. Under the spectrum of detrimental you have radiation and microwaves. These are damaging wavelengths from electrical fields such as those emitted from cell phones, fluorescent lighting, computers, smoke detectors and the more recent and ever popular "Wi-Fi." Keep in mind that "Wi-Fi," once directed and aimed at your home or neighborhood, can not be turned off.

The Fluorescent Factor

Canada is now in the process of phasing out incandescent lighting and so is the United States, which sounds like just the promising "green" change that environmentalists were looking for. Indeed, many are rejoicing over these compact glass gadgets that have been hailed as money/energy earth savers. Why is the fact that

CFL's are filled with mercury, emit microwaves, are labeled a biohazard that let off a strong and dangerous electromagnetic field being virtually ignored or downplayed in almost every article touting its "benefits"? With these serious health implications to consider, it is worth it for our society to take a deeper look at the CFL phenomena and what its potential impact on the human race might be. Let us not forget what the impact that nuclear energy has already left on our entire world; a technology that was also once esteemed as a monetary and environmental breakthrough by many of the same organizations that are pushing the fluorescent lighting agenda today.

So what light should we use? Obviously, the most perfect source would be the sun itself, (yes, the sun, you know that big bright ball in the sky that has accumulated so many enemies these days?). You may be thinking that I am going to tell you that I use a full-spectrum light, LEDs, or halogen…but think again.

Non-frosted, clear, incandescent bulbs, hands down, best mimic the spectrum of natural sunlight. Does that surprise you? This is probably because you have been lied to for so long about the benefits of "full-spectrum" lighting. A full-spectrum light or "Ott-light" is a bulb that has had the color yellow completely removed from its spectrum (Dinshah, 2005). Taking out the yellow makes everything appear clearer and crisper, however, the fact that the color blue is completely missing is creates a potential imbalance to the human body. A regular non-frosted incandescent bulb has a larger amount of yellow than natural sunlight; however it has a complete spectrum and is not missing any colors. Even with my rejection of the Ott light and the full-spectrum light, do not think that I disregard the work of John Ott, the founder of full-spectrum lighting. To the contrary, Dr. Ott's research on the dangers of fluorescent lighting on the human body and environment is a powerful voice of dissent among the hypnotized masses. His pioneering research 25 years ago on the biological effects of light sources on the human body is as relevant today as it was then.

We no longer need to rely solely on Ott's work for information about the dangers of fluorescent lighting. Robert

Brennan from the New York Megaphone recently wrote an article calling for the removal of fluorescent lighting from public work places, schools and businesses. Brennan states that fluorescent lighting causes mental and physical illness and poses risks to people who live and work under the lights all day long (Brennan, 2007). Citing revolutionary research from such well-regarded scientists and researchers as Dr. Richard Stevens, an epidemiologist from the University of Connecticut Medical Center and Laurence Martel, the Ph.D president of the National Academy of integrated learning, Brennan makes an irrefutable case against the "environmentally un-friendly" fluorescent lighting.

Fluorescent lighting has been linked to illnesses plaguing our society today, such as depression, leukemia, melanoma, anxiety, tooth decay, sleep disorders, headaches, SAD, and aggressive behavior. New studies have now proven that people who worked outdoors in the sun all day had the lowest amounts of skin cancer while office workers who worked under fluorescent lights all day had the highest (Cousens, 2000).

Protecting Our Children from the Fluorescent Fallout

While shopping at a home improvement store in 2007, I noticed a man knock down a stand of at least 15 fluorescent lights. Startled by the loud crash, I turned around to see what fell and immediately sought out my children to keep them away from the biohazard "spill". In the midst of the chaos, several employees dashed over to pick up the pieces of glass with bare hands. One employee was merely sweeping it up into a dustpan. Customers, oblivious to the mercury and carcinogenic danger, simply stepped over and onto the debris.

I already knew about the perils of the fluorescent clean up protocol, having just read about the plight of a woman from Prospect, Maine named Brandy Bridges who had a fluorescent bulb break in her child's bedroom. Ms. Bridges contacted Home Depot, the store who sold her the bulb. They warned her not to simply vacuum up the broken bulb and go about her day, but to immediately call the poison control. What ensued in the following months was a dangerous fiasco that falls short of a home-based reality show called "Biohazard Survivors". She was instructed to completely seal off her child's bedroom after the room tested above safe levels for mercury and then, to hire a company that cleans up mercury spills for no less than $2,000! She also found out that her home insurance would not pay for such a service (Farah, 2007). This leads me to ask a personal question to fellow American's everywhere: How many people do you know return burnt out CFL's to the store for disposal? How many people do you know have cleaned up fluorescent bulbs with their bare hands and a vacuum cleaner, completely oblivious to the dangers?

  This emphasizes the gravity of my shock at the way the store handled this. Furthermore, I imagined children running over to that same area and touching and playing on the ground where the spill occurred. I went to two different managers and received a different answer from each one. The first, manager told me that there was no danger as chemicals simply "evaporate" into the air upon breaking. The second manager explained the protocol that it uses is in accordance to HAZMAT, OSHA, and EPA guidelines when cleaning up. This involves reporting the spill, wearing special gloves to handle materials, and disposing the gloves with the broken CFLs. This is followed by the thorough spraying of a special solution and sealing off the area from customers until the clean-up is over. This manager seemed disappointed by his employees disregard for biohazard protocol but was not immediately alarmed either. This led me to write to make several phone calls seeking answers which all lead nowhere. I now believe because of the marriage between CFLs, special interest groups, and government agencies, it can only be up to the American public to educate themselves and protect their families from this potential environmental catastrophe.

  The fact that Germany has already restricted the use of fluorescent lighting in public places and has banned fluorescent lights in hospitals shows us that this issue is too great to be shrugged off and ignored (Brennan). We should follow Germany's path instead of Canada's in regards to lighting and start as a country looking at more relevant and pressing issues that are beckoning for our attention. Clean water and the effects of fluoride, pesticides and insecticides on our health and water table—these are all things that are spiraling out of control and that we have to begin taking seriously. While climate change has been a part of life on earth for millions of years, the utter and complete destruction of our environment through man-made chemicals has not.

Food, Vitamins and Supplements

Real food quality has been difficult to obtain and monitor objectively because the government has attempted to take over the organic food industry. There are farmers who refuse to get an FDA organic certification on their untreated cows because they consider the standards the government has set to be too low! Companies like Coca Cola and Nestle are buying out organic food companies. It is important now more than ever to begin to stand by our organic American farmers who resist mass-produced, genetically-modified garbage. These men and women are the true freedom fighters and they are championing for the health and protection of the entire human race.

Many people have said, "Western medicine has provided the answers that the earth couldn't for thousands of years." They will also say, "Look at all the people who died of polio without the vaccine, or the bubonic plague, and people didn't live very long in times before." Before what, I ask? We have to look back before the Crusades and Inquisition, when knowledge of health and healing was a crime. For the last 2,000 years health, healing, and even the natural functions of our bodies have been treated as closely guarded secrets. We had to buy our health from the religious hierarchy the same way we do now with the medical community. Religion and politics has manipulated and coerced health and healing for over four thousand years. We are now, only within the last 50 years, been allowed to practice healing ourselves and to have access to, ultimately, our own being.

There is a flipside to becoming more health-conscious, however. We too easily risk falling into hypnotic schemes that persuade us to lose control of our health again. We can get lost in the gamut of expensive vitamins and pills and lose sight of the basic principles that underlie these supplements to health and well-being. People who are searching for healing need to start at the core by learning to trust and listen to themselves; to stop buying into the high-pressure sales tactics for products that may not be beneficial. The health industry is severely manipulated, like every other industry. Let's face it; there are some people who will spend their entire lives trying to make a million dollars dishonestly off an unsuspecting population. Those people are hoping and praying that you will just trust them instead of yourself.

Whenever the message you hear or read declares that "you need this [product] to live" or "without this $30 vitamin-herb combination you will die," consider it a red flag, even when you start to feel that way without necessarily "hearing" it. These messages do as much damage to the self as allopathic medicine does. They accomplish little more than creating a race of "healthy" individuals that believe they are healthy as long as they invest and take "their pills." No. We want to get away from the money-making mind schemes by turning off our access to advertisements, whether these occur in the proliferation of so called "health magazines" or in the media.

Balance is imperative. We have to be careful not to hurt our bodies with obsessive-compulsive health ideals. Many people will eat that hamburger they have been craving, all the while thinking, "this is making me fat, I shouldn't be eating this." Or they could be smoking a cigarette and thinking "this is killing me." Similarly, some will experience panic and anxiety if they do not have a daily dose of their "wonder pills." These confusing thoughts actually damage the self and retard any hope for healing and growth. There needs to be a time of introspection and protection --first to heal, and then to strengthen. The result of this is the emergence of the spirit from the cocoon of life, as the real person, fully expressed, unveiled and ready to soar.

Ayurveda: Something Healing for Everyone

As a committed yoga practitioner, I eventually found myself in the midst of Ayurveda, which is the most ancient science of natural healing from India. Its basic tenet is that everyone is fire, water, or air. The Ayurvedic treatments are as simple as adding a few spices and as complex as staying at a facility for a total body detoxification. It is similar to Chinese medicine, which is also elemental in nature but far less comprehensive. Given what I knew before I encountered it, Ayurveda made sense to me. Subsequently, I searched out a local Ayurvedic doctor for myself.

The doctor I went to see was 40 miles from my home and was recommended by a friend; an added bonus was that she was covered by my insurance because she was also a medical doctor. She was very nice and was from India, the birthplace of the practice. At the beginning of our session, she gave me a pulse diagnosis and then recommended some herbs from Maharishi™ Ayurveda. I was diagnosed with a water imbalance (a kapha dosha) and was advised to drink lassis (herbal yogurt drink), exercise, and take some water-decreasing Maharishi herbs.

I took all the herbs and followed all of my recommendations. I kept getting sicker and sicker and bigger and bigger (I was 30 lbs overweight). I was beginning to lose faith in Ayurveda, but by this time, was studying it independently and could see the main flaw with my treatment, which lasted about eight months. I had all three doshas (the physical constitutions of fire, water, and air) severely excessed. I was filled with mucus, which is water, I was constipated, which is air, and had skin breakouts, which is fire. By all Ayurvedic standards, I was considered terminal and chronic and would need the intense detoxification process called Pancha Karma.

Pancha Karma takes anywhere from a few weeks to a few months. You often go and stay at an Ayurvedic facility where you are attended to by many people with different specialties. In a nutshell, the treatment consists of dosha specific meals, oils, herbs, massages, enemas (bastis), etc. At this time I was in school studying naturopathy and Ayurveda and I also had three small children, so going to stay at a facility was out of the question for me at that time. I spent many months experimenting and creating a Pancha Karma treatment facility within my home environment. This also later evolved into the Aurore Method, which I will expound on later.

An important facet of Ayurveda is always taking an herb with dosha-appropriate carriers. A carrier basically takes the herbs to different tissues and layers in the body. A carrier can be yogurt, sucanat, honey, oils, or ghee, the decision between these depends on your excessed dosha. This is an essential part of getting the nutrients deep into the system and organs. This practice is also missing from many modern naturopathic practices. In Ayurveda there has to be a mixture of tastes and any too much of one taste could be detrimental. For instance, a little yogurt is good, but it can be too heavy, sweet, sour and cold. Too much yogurt can actually clog your shrotas (system) and keep your body from properly metabolizing.

Ayurveda and the Orgone

I discovered an important link between Ayurveda and Orgonomy. It was the ability of Orgone therapy to change dosha. When I started my Orgone treatment, I had a water imbalance, which had exaggerated my weight and also kept me sick and filled with mucus. My personality was also water, which means I was very laid back and easy going. I was lacking energy and was always tired. However, shortly after my Orgonomy treatments, I came to have an air imbalance. Not only was I severely constipated, I also found myself suffering from bouts of "air" trapped in my intestines (gas pain). An interesting product of this was that my personality changed dramatically; I was bursting with energy but it came in the form of incessant worrying, and acting on edge, shaky, and nervousness. I started having anxiety and panic attacks. After a few months of this I went on to a fire imbalance which led to diarrhea, acne, and feelings of anger. I felt like I could fly off the handle at any moment. Rage is what I felt inside. Being innately aware of my body and feelings by doing self-experimentation, I logged my experiences in a journal. I found that, amazingly, my dosha had changed three times in a year.

This led me to come to the conclusion that we are all hypothetically born with a primary dosha of fire, and have either water or air tendencies. I know this doesn't fit into the ideal configuration, but let me explain. If you study karma outside of past life debt and bring it into the present life you can see how it fits together nicely. For example, I can look at an astrology chart and see how the planets relate to an individual's health (this practice is called Jyotish and is one aspect of Ayurveda). I can say these problems are attributed to a past life, and while this is debatable for some, I can prove their present life karma with their family and what they came into and what they need to overcome. This is without any mystical pretense but just by questioning people about their childhood and present health.

This is where science and spirituality merge. This is where the intangible becomes provable. You can choose to approach sickness and disease mystically, which does not seem to be a powerful enough catalyst for change for the individual, or you can approach it a bit more scientifically and a bit more in the here and now. We have to approach life with what we experience as real and tangible. Everybody can benefit from prayer, but when it comes to becoming honest and raising our levels of conscious awareness, we need to be careful how far out of earth and into heaven we go. I say that only because escapism via mysticism or spirituality can be dangerous if it keeps you from evolving, from getting well, from being able to see truth.

Orgonomy teaches the importance of the organism's ability to express all ranges of feeling and emotion. As small children, our divine right to exist is severely thwarted and changed by individuals who step into our life from many areas—parents, school, religion, government, media. These forces break down and suppress all aspects of our personality simply because it was done to them.

That is the true circle of karma. Many individuals on this planet will, in fact, hate their parents for a time and will even resist them but eventually become just like them. Guilt and shame are strong culprits and are introduced to the child in-utero. Put as simply as possible, the child is born into the parents' pain and reality.

The Fire Within

A fire or pitta personality is one that is able to express anger. Some fire personalities will say they know they are angry or have an anger problem. This is the opposite trait to a water personality, who will carry their anger within and will often deny even being angry. Many fire personalities will spend their entire lives trying to put out the fire that is part of their nature. Perhaps this is because they are afraid that their turbulent emotions will grow out of control. When these fire personalities explode they can scare themselves and others and as many of us come to understand a fire personality, they have certainly been known to go too far at times.

I come from a different perspective. I pose this question: "Is having and expressing anger wrong?" Most of us are deathly afraid of people who express anger in any form. Is that the angry person's fault or is it actually our personal perspective on anger? Anger is one (of many) human emotions that is not tolerated very well by others. Many water personalities may have started life as a fire personality but following a series of parental interventions, such as spankings, shaming and rejection, the person's ability to express themselves goes underground. Many water constitutions will feel the anger starting to stir (while they typically cannot admit or recognize this) and will eat to subdue their emotions. Just as our culture does not tolerate anger from children, they certainly do not tolerate people who are overweight. Yet many of these overweight people are by-products of being raised in a culture and family where they were forced to subdue and repress anger.

When someone admits they are angry, even without showing any signs of aggression, they elicit a negative response from the people around them. Others will challenge their feelings instead of just letting them exist. "You have no right to be angry" is a standard (not natural) response. Another reaction to anger is, "You're angry, well, I am the one that should be angry!!" These response are contemptuous and make most people feel they are not allowed to be or feel anger at all. When someone can actually arrive at the point where they can admit their emotion, others may actually feel jealous and possibly enraged. The other person can be taken back psychologically to childhood where they are kicking and screaming: "Let me be angry, too!"

The air personality can be described as nervous energy, or someone with "too many eggs in one basket." An air personality will have a conversation with you and will switch topics often without a cue. They can suffer from bouts of paranoia and intense worrying. Their incessant worrying and often unfounded fears is often an over-exaggerated attempt to cover up repressed, deep-seated emotion. Many air personalities are known for their obsessive-compulsive traits or habits. This is an effort that the organism continually makes to try to establish and maintain sanity or a comfort level by placing grave importance on small things. This means that they do not have to look at or feel the "real thing" that is actually eating away at them.

Ayurveda teaches that all of us have a little of all three doshas, but we are actually primarily directed by two. I differ from ancient precepts of Ayurveda when it lays blame primarily on diet and past-life karma. To a degree, I suppose this is merely a case of semantics, but I feel the importance, again, has to be placed on the here and now. Many of us are trying to recover from traumatic childhoods, without knowing how or even why we do what we do. Hence, the reason why I use the term *karma* to convey the importance of the soul's present life circumstance.

We need to overcome many of these obstinate negative behaviors, not just in preparation for our next life, but also for our children and their children's children. It is too easy to blame our present health and condition on sin, spiritual warfare, or past-life events. The fact is, we all have the ability to change and we all have the *right* to be healthy Let us stop putting obstacles in our way and start accepting our right to be healed.

Drowning in a Watery Grave

I had assumed I was a water personality since birth, but Orgonomy had shown me that I truly was not who I thought I was. When I started finding my feelings, accepting them without guilt, and getting the feelings physically out of my body by hitting inanimate objects, I finally began to lose weight. The release was absolutely necessary. I had three small children that tried my patience and brought me to the brink of love, hate and aspects of all human emotions every day. I would find I would wake up angry before my children even got out of bed. I would go in my bedroom and get all of my negative feelings out on my pillow and then start the day out right with my children.

As a water personality, I did not spank the children as much as I rejected them for their anger and mine. When the anger started to build, I would hang out in the kitchen eating and ignore my children by talking on the phone. Other times, I would lie on the couch in a state of dire depression, a state that might have been exacerbated by the deep fear I had about expressing anger to my children or even just feeling it in the first place. I would nap and they would play around me. I would go in and out of my motherhood throughout the day. Reading them a story and then becoming so emotionally exhausted and stressed from contact that I was practically passing out on the couch.

In Orgonomy, I dealt with my childhood experience of having a water mother and a fire father. My father was dominant and militant—he was the only one in the house allowed to be angry. If we even showed an expression on our face that we were angry, our expression would be met with swift and severe punishment. I realized that most of the human emotion I started to experience was always hampered and filtered through survival mechanisms such as fear of rejection, shame for being a female, and guilt for feeling anything at all. This created who I was, something I was not able to understand fully until much later in my life.

The point is, we need to realize the combination of innate personality traits and those of our parents (and the effects of that mixture) while communicating with others. Whether we are confronting others with anger, or "constructive criticism" we need to be honestly aware of our motives and how we are coming across to people. Again, this brings us back to intention and perception. Actively realizing and working through these painful aspects of my personality allowed me to change my dosha, and more importantly, to change my life.

No Anger Welcomed Here

Why are angry people looked at as misfits in our culture? In fact, I venture to say that the fire/anger person is closer to ultimate health mentally and physically than anyone else. The only problem they truly have is twofold: 1), how they express their anger (which is usually to the detriment of others), and 2) the guilt and anguish they experience after having expressed it. These people usually are forced by others—be it by law enforcement or by loved ones—to go to "anger management" courses. A fire personality will try to stifle the brewing emotions with liquor or drugs. This is an effort the fire personalities make to subdue them selves and try to control their behavior. (Ayurveda actually calls liquor "fire water," which inevitably will make them more fire.)

You eventually see the fire come out on their skin, through acne because it builds up and stores in their liver. The liver and kidneys back up and the impurities are let out into the blood and onto the skin. A more advanced case of such fire symptoms will be acid indigestion, gout, and crippling inflammatory conditions such as back problems or fire in the joints. When the fire or repressed anger gets to this level, the organism basically starts turning on itself and attacking itself. The joints and vertebrae are severely compressed by the tense muscles and ligaments. Literally, their movement is compromised and painful.

The fire person has the choice of loading up on antacids, medicated creams, and painkillers. Naturopathically, they can take enzymes to eat up the acid and inflammation and herbs to calm them, like Valerian and St. John's Wort. Ayurvedically, they can take rose tea with mint and do yoga and breathing exercises. All of these different methods are efforts to control the fire. But what about the innate needs of the fire personalities to release their pent up rage? People who are fire personalities need to release their anger from time to time, no matter how much yoga or herbs they take or psychotherapy they may have. Talking is inferior to the aspect of physically working it out of the body. Have you have ever heard the saying, "there are people who talk and people who do?" People realize that talking never stops and often can lead to further stifling repression.

Unfortunately, when the fire releases anger it will likely be followed by judgment, shame, and guilt from everyone involved with the fire personality. I have taught my fire clients, or my clients that get to the fire stage, to actively hit something inanimate—to get their rage out on something that feels no pain before it builds to an uncontrollable level. If they can at least get to the point where they can recognize how they are feeling, they are on the road to wellness. Being able to admit love, fear, hate, or sadness *without guilt* is very important. People need to let go of their conditioned, often moral-based, beliefs about anger and work proactively with their body and emotions to release the fire when nature calls them to do so.

Recognizing who or what they are angry at is also very important. They are not just hitting to hit, but actually going through and releasing the emotional aspects as well. This is the part that essentially frees them and allows them to heal. I tell my children that when the hatred and anger come out, the love and happiness comes in. It is a circle of energy and emotion. And in this circle, this cycle, there is no guilt and no shame.

It's All About Contact and the Elements

A fire person pushes people away with their critical, judgmental nature; a water person will push people away with their excess weight and lethargy; an air person will push others away by their inability to follow through and their much ungrounded, exaggerated perception of others and themselves. The importance here is to look at and realize that all of our dosha/personality imbalances severely thwart our ability to make human contact. This is a primary aspect to any healing regimen. When we can make eye contact with another human being, we can reach out and touch and be touched; this can be painful, but yet healing in and of itself.

In a society that is noteworthy for its lack of human contact and honest human emotion, many of us are suffering, if not dying, from this phenomenon of emotional denial. Trust is an essential goal and has to be actively sought. But how do we trust when we had parents, teachers, and doctors we could not trust? We came into the world trusting, so the real problem is that we have been taught or conditioned not to trust.

Perhaps this is one of the reasons why some Americans are comfortable hiding out in a world where only God can help them and only God can heal them. They act as if they trust no one but God. The reality is they are alone here on earth (I speak of human contact and not spiritual right now). Many of these people will die isolated and alone, just like the Beatles' song "Eleanor Rigby." They may be surrounded at that time by plenty of people they know, but no one that they trust.

The moral for me is simple: when I was a zealously religious person I pushed a lot of people away from me and somehow, I was always sick. My heart hardened toward everyone and I was living in hate, even though I proclaimed love. If I had remained in that environment I probably would have wound up in with a life-threatening disease. Instead, I left that environment, left the harmful belief system, which proved to be a lot more difficult then just leaving a building. This is how I found healing and love, for me, for my family and now for others. In essence, I had to leave the harsh, judgmental reality I was living in to heal and experience true compassion. Up until then, my life was just an empty religious façade, rehearsed and devoid of genuine feeling.

The Ayurvedic texts speak of the importance for every person to recognize the divine light or "God" within themselves, that they are literally a part of God. For an Atheist, it is about helping them understand the power and energy within and not offending them with religious rhetoric. For a Christian, this should be as simple reading about Jesus teachings (the red letters in their bibles) and applying it faithfully to their lives. Teachings on loving and accepting others present a concept that is virtually ignored in the Church, but should take years to study, expound on, and to apply to our lives. Ayurveda asserts that our disconnection from divinity is the main underlying emotional problem buried beneath cancer and sickness (Tirtha, 1998). Truly we must examine what and who our God is, be it Jesus, Krishna, Allah or the Sun and Moon. If your God is not a God of love and acceptance, then the belief is hurting you more than it is helping you.

This is the main problem I found with the alternative holistic cancer books I had to read for school. They spent much time talking about poison foods, poison chemicals in our homes. etc. When it came to the emotional aspects of cancer, all of the cancer books I had read fell short. This is because when it came to the subject of repressed emotions, the books sought to moralize feelings and sought to encourage individuals to further repress their feelings. This creates guilty feelings among individuals and guilt for just being human. Guilt and shame are major contributing factors in any illness.

There is an Ayurvedic book on cancer called, "The Answer to Cancer" by Sharma, Mishra and Meade. This is a light-hearted, often humorous book on cancer, which seems impossible—and perhaps that is where one of its strengths lies. I liked the helpful Ayurvedic recommendations it gave but I found the sarcastic tone to be too indirect and confusing. The book was educating until the authors attempted to "religious-ize" the book. The authors actually refer to anger as a negative "behavior" that needs to be stopped. Another behavior that they say needs to be stopped is hate (Sharma, Mishra and Meade, 2002). I can use myself as an example and say, I am a human and I experience a full range of human emotions and feelings. These include love and hate, happiness and sadness, and anger and passion. Physically expressing any human emotion in a healthy manner is necessary for any health program. I am not talking about getting angry and kicking a car in that is too close to your car but about an actual allowing of self-expression. Kicking or hitting your bed when you feel hatred or anger—hugging or making love to someone when you feel love or passion. This inevitably goes back to the cliché, "get real."

The New-Age vs. Orgonomy

In a previous chapter I eluded to the contradictory nature of the New Age movements and many of its advocates. The example I will provide for you is the very well known and very "loving" Louise Hay. She is a writer, lecturer and cancer survivor. Many of my clients talk about her philosophy and her books. They seem to really enjoy the premise of her books, which is basically that loving and forgiving everyone is essential to good health. I read Louise Hay's book, *You Can Heal Your Life*. I will agree that it is a beautiful book filled with lots of flowers, hearts, and pretty birds. Louise shares her personal story of tremendous childhood trauma and how she overcame cancer. She has written a very warm and fuzzy book about how to overcome horrendous circumstances and also, heal your body. Her simple approach to healing sounds good and even feels good to read about.

Despite these heartwarming aspects that are innately appealing, let me further expound on what Louise Hay is teaching others. She wrote 247 pages about loving, accepting and forgiving. She speaks about how resentment can make a person sick, but describes it in terms of damaging thought processes that can be changed easily within the moment. She says that, "New thought patterns (positive affirmations) can heal and relax your body." She even goes into grave detail about each sickness and what emotions are connected with it. A sinus infection, for example, is someone you are trying to block out. Acne, Louise says, responds to telling yourself "I am wonderful" (Hay, 1999). On page 20 I read, "I have found that forgiving and releasing resentment will dissolve even cancer". On page 21 she says, "One must *dissolve resentment* when it is easy and not wait until you are under the surgeons' knife". About now, you should be wondering how Louise directs one to "release and dissolve" resentment, saying "we need to choose to release the past and forgive everyone." She follows this premise throughout the book, repeating this philosophy later by recommending that we "Stay away from thoughts that create problems and pain."

One may assume by the gilded pages and the beautiful words in the book that Louise Hay dissolved her cancer by not thinking any damaging thoughts--easily and miraculously forgiving everyone, even herself. Well, I thought this too, all the way up until near the conclusion where she describes how she *really* overcame cancer. Here is how she describes it in her own words, "With the help of a good therapist, I expressed all of the old, bottled-up anger by beating pillows and howling with rage".

Hmmh, sounds like Louise Hay had some rage-releasing Orgonomy treatments! Why then would she waste our time (sorry to all of the people on the "Hayride") with all of this; fluffy, pretty, beat around the bush advice? I don't think Louise even realizes how misleading and contradictory her book is. A whole book written on the importance of dissolving resentment-without getting into the very important question of How? Perhaps, she has disassociated that very important part of her healing journey or maybe got scared that the truth would not "sell".

Her philosophy is to just "love" and that love heals and uses her own life as an example. However, I question even her ability to actually do so. She admits to giving a child away birth and never reaching out and reconciling the relationship with that child. In this case, I believe the word love is substituted for the action of avoidance. Eventually, these avoidance/feel good tactics are self-deprecating and that aspect would eventually come to the readers mind. She eventually looses people with her mystical feel good approach. Of course, there will always be people that hang around just to try to convince others that they have reached the impossible point of loving and forgiving by chanting magical words and erasing thoughts. A holier than thou attitude will both isolate and win them many followers. I argue that even then, the charade must eventually come to an end, and one day they will need to also: Get Real and feel.

The New-Age Land of Oz

Louise's information on her body-mind connection is "metaphysically" based. The truth is, Reich and Ellsworth Baker had done all of the body and mind research over 50 years ago. Even though Hay alludes to having gone through Orogonomy treatments, she never once recognized Reich's research or call it "Orgonomy". In one paragraph of her book she mentions body work. Amazingly, she actually recommends Rolfing but also mentions Bioenergetics as opposed to Orgonomy. Her "Orgonomy" story that she mentions in her biography was nothing like a bioenergetic session. What was she afraid of? I don't know, but Louise Hay touches on a subject that is much, much more deep and complex than just textbook affirmations. To say that one's stomach problems arise from not digesting information takes away from the depth and complexity of the body and mind. In fact, it is such an over-simplification that it is almost offensive.

New Age life recommendations expect you to start at point A which is non-awareness, move to point B which is awareness, and then arrive spontaneously at point Z without going through necessary steps along the way. They opt to avoid the "hard" stuff and focus on the love "fluff". Where would Dorothy be had she not taken the yellow brick road to get to Oz? On the yellow brick road there was a complete balance of good and bad characters and experiences. Even the witches were divided into two good and two bad.

So, what about other New Age "metaphysical" authors and speakers? Well, I have found Carolyn Myss's information to be slightly more intriguing. I am referring to her double CD, *Why People Don't Heal*. She talks about mystics, but can also openly admit that she doesn't know any and has only read about them. She also says that life affirmations and positive thinking won't work unless the perception has been "activated". Myss falls short when she describes how to activate perception for life change and fizzles out into a sort of nonsensical rant with many, many steps and ideas that are tedious and actually just boil down to the same thing we've all heard before-- positive thinking and life affirmations. After listening to her CD, I was left feeling confused and stressed. Let me get this right, I am supposed to activate my perception to be healed, so that life affirmations can work using life affirmations?

Wounded Children

I am very focused on the importance of the parent/child relationship and bringing the two together. Myss describes teen angst as being caused from parents being intimidated by their children. This offended me because I was once a teenager and my angst was legitimate. The most healing, life-changing experience at that time would have been my parents coming to me and admitting their faults and reaching out. This would have brought us to a heartfelt level and would have placed my parents in a life-affirming role. It would have taken them out of the "hypocrisy" pile that I had put them in. As a teenager, I was sick of all of the fake emptiness in the universe. I was longing for a heartfelt connection with something in the world.

What to Do with Old Wounds?

"Woundology" is a term coined by Myss. She says that we are all connecting to each other through our pain simply by going around and telling people, "I was abused" or "I was beaten" and that we need to stop. She makes a startling, poignant observation when she describes survivor groups and psychotherapy as a boat that people take to get to the other side of their experience. She goes on to say that these survivors get stuck on the boat and never get off on the other side. I loved that metaphor and she is highly accurate in her assessment of victimization. However, I believe that many people are greatly unaware of their feelings and chronically and hurriedly trying to hide abuse and their past. Many people try to connect on a superficial level by avoiding their core and talking about *other people's pain* (avoiding their own). This stands in sharp contrast to sharing painful life truths and reaching out from a deeper heartfelt level.

Three Levels of Disconnection

I feel that Myss might be reaching out to 5-30% of the population with the woundology theory. We all know someone who is constantly dwelling on and nursing old wounds. In light of this, any person at any given level of healing or awareness is in danger of disconnecting and could miss the connection level altogether. They then *pretend* to have arrived at point Z but they are really still stagnating at point C.

The general idea is that most of this information lacks a heartfelt connection and is stuck in the head or on an intellectual level. This is true no matter how *spiritual* people try to make it. The problem is avoiding contact with the self and each other. I offer you several examples of disconnection from several levels of awareness:

- Level 1- I go around and tell everyone I am fine and cover up my pain with beautiful clothes, make-up, and narcissist lies- result: disconnection, alienation, isolation.

- Level 2- I go around and tell everyone I am a survivor of abuse and have been abused-result: disconnection, alienation, isolation.

Being honest about wounding is one thing, but often the connection to the pain through the heart is not there. How do you go around and tell people you were severely abused without tears, anguish, or feeling in your face? These people are not truly connected to the pain and anger and are using their wounds for entertainment purposes only.

- Level 3- I go around and tell everyone I have made it through abuse and I am enlightened now. I spend my time trying to convince others, including myself, that all I had to do is meditate, pray, and pretend there was no pain—no negative feelings. That my old wounds magically disappeared and all of my hate was turned into love.

Result: more disconnection, alienation, isolation but also adoration and naïve followers.

I feel like this is the worst type because they are playing with the religious/Darwin type ideas that they are "special" people—that they are on the top and only the strong survive. This borders on mental abuse because of the use of "god" language, often tied to the power of suggestion. For more information on this read the classic fable "The Emperors New Clothes" by Hans Christian Anderson.

My Point of View

A 35-year-old man came to see me to help cure chronic migraine headaches. After several consultations and herbal recommendations, I found out that he had had a traumatic experience after migrating to the U.S. from Iraq. A male friend once told him to be circumcised or else the American women will find him "weird or gross". Following this advice he got the circumcision and lost most of the sensation in his penis. He was in touch with his anger, which showed he was farther on his journey than others. However, he was stuck in a support group for men recovering from circumcision. This turned out to be a sedentary victim hate group instead of a catalyst for change. I told him he needed to make the journey out of this group and seek out Orgonomy treatments to get to the reason of his headaches. This man looked shocked and even fearful. After our consultation, he spoke to the group director about me and then never contacted me again.

The director of the anti-circumcision group had been stuck in his rage for more than 20 years. To his credit, he is a good man and one of the leading advocates against infant circumcision. It is his anger and connection with his wounds that fuels his activism. He is, quite visibly, an intensely unhappy man. However, he is also still an important societal force for change. This is often the heart of activism that can and will make the person sick. Pain is their power and they use it to accomplish great things. They are suffering from <u>not</u> physically getting the rage out of their body and not crying through the pain. They hold it in, churn it, feed it and then explode through activist means. In fairness to Myss and Hay, the "love affirmations" may take the anger/sadness based victims far *after* they had worked sufficiently through their rage and sadness.

Life Affirmations and Positive Thinking Will Work!

It is not my intentions to make you feel that positive thinking is a waste of time. For someone who grew up in a well-balanced family and did not experience a lot of psychological trauma and neurosis, positive thinking might be just the thing to pull you out of a rut. Then, there is the severely traumatized group. These are people who have been savagely beaten, used, tortured sexually, and psychologically damaged. For these people, it may be too much for them physically and psychologically go back and release the abuse. These people have survived because of their ability to disassociate and mentally escape. I am not saying they are hopeless but the positive thinking stuff might be as heavy as they will ever go.

Last year, a woman wanted me to treat her for allergies, headaches and depression. Initially, I learned her husband died when she was newly married with two children and that she was now in a relationship with a man that was abusing her. Finally, she told me that she had been a foster child and was sexually abused by several different foster fathers. She explained that the angels brought her through it and that she often goes to the "angel" place.

I knew that I was not qualified to bring her through her pain or sickness at that time. I will use constitutional homeopathy with the my own method but it has to be within certain parameters. I could clearly see this woman needed this armor and defense; I did not want to touch it or challenge her on it. To activate her perception for healing (a term used by Myss) I would need to take her through the other side of the water and connect her body and mind. Everyone deserves healing, but I recognized that within my capacity and training, I could not be the one. So, I urged her to go to Rolfing sessions or get Orgonomy treatments before I saw her.

Yoga and Orgone: A Marriage of Give and Take

A few years ago, I found myself (finally) in an advanced form of yoga during which I was strong and flexible. After Orgonomy, however, my body changed and locked up in various parts. I especially found plough pose (laying down with feet and legs straight above and over my head) to change dramatically with each Orgonomy session. Whether it was because of my upper back by my shoulders, or my middle and lower back, my ability to fully stretch was hindered.

This did not discourage me; rather, it enlightened me as to how energy flowed and damned up within my system. While it appeared to be physically hampering my body, what was actually taking place was that the emotional pain and trauma held deep in my bodily organs were making their way to the surface, the muscular system. The energy can only go out, expand, and be released or it can be smothered and stuffed back in, to cause disease. I used a combination of intentional hitting and yoga and kept experimenting until I came up with my own Aurore yoga. This type of yoga uses mouth breathing instead of nose breathing, and deep emotional release. I created this out of my belief that the organism should be able to start or continue freeing itself up from deep emotional pain (although I never advocate replacing Orgone therapy, which is primary).

I wanted to give the millennial public something they could embrace, learn, carry and teach. I wanted every individual to have access to their true selves and their true identity. The fact that yoga has emerged as a mainstream form of exercise is exciting. All people who study yoga, spiritually or not, know about the emotional thresholds that yoga can take you to. Getting into a certain pose can sometimes generate tears and intense emotional responses. Many of us, if we are in a class, will hold back those tears and dismiss the feelings deep within our bodies that are desperately trying to reach the surface. This is partly because the organism wants to heal itself. Your body cries out from within and sends you messages everyday. Yoga is your effort at meeting those messages halfway.

Other times, instead of crying, when people meet the pivotal emotional points in their yoga practice, they become scared and release their pose. The problem then is not that the person lacks the bodily strength to hold the pose, but that they suddenly find they lack the emotional strength to endure it. We reach the apex we so actively sought, but at the peak, we turn back out of fear.

We are simply afraid to feel. The foundations of this fear are simple; we were raised in a society that has taught us it is wrong. Raised in a society that tells us emotions are not safe, that we cannot trust our emotions. Often, it is our emotional body that cries out first and then many years later our physical body follows suit. Instead of crying, we lose our eyesight and hair; instead of breathing, we have heart attacks and asthma.

The pelvis is always a touchy part of the body for many people. That is the part of our body where we hold the most emotional pain. Many people have been abused in their pelvic area in someway, be it through rape or circumcision. The pelvis is always the last segment in the body to be worked on in Orgonomy. Releasing your tears, your aggression and your breath is a good place to start.

Naturopathy and Ayurveda

There are many aspects of health that Ayurveda introduces that Naturopathy often glosses over. I spoke of the herb carriers as one, but there is another: the conflict between herbs and dosha. To see the difference, consider the herb pau d'arco used for yeast/candida infections. This is one herb prescribed by many herbalists and naturopaths to overcome systemic yeast or compromised immunity. The problem with this recommendation is that pau d'arco is a cooling herb. If you have a water/kapha or air/vata dosha and are taking this herb for yeast, you can be assured that you are not helping your yeast infection and will probably be making it worse.

As an Ayurvedic Doctor of Natural Health I would only recommend pau d'arco to someone who was a fire/pitta dosha and was presenting symptoms of yeast on their skin. Most of the people with systemic yeast infections are dealing with air and water problems. This is because the excess air in their systems has caused their intestines to become dry, therefore leading to constipation. This in turn causes a water excess as mucus and allergic responses build up in the system because it is getting "backed up." The yeast and parasites live inside the mucus and thrive off the compacted fecal matter. All of this adds up to a person that needs warming spices to start breaking down the mucus and release the compacted fecal matter.

Typical naturopaths will keep their candida patients on a steady dose of herbs, probiotics, and enzymes. Some of these herbs include addictive herbs affecting the colon, using cascara sagrada or senna as laxatives. You will find quite a few natural health practitioners continually taking herbal laxatives because the peristalsis activity in their intestines has been severely compromised and they have lost the ability to "move their bowels."

Many naturopaths also recommend colonics to help breakdown the buildup of fecal matter. While an occasional colonic may be useful, in Ayurveda, it is not recommended because the water colonic is too drying for an air/constipated individual. The colonic may initially help to break down mucus, but it then introduces more dryness to the colon, thereby exacerbating constipating air qualities. In contrast, I only recommend dosha-appropriate herbal enemas to my clients with dosha-correlating color on the pelvis and mid-section. An example would be to use mixture of licorice, dashmula (Indian herbs) and sesame oil and the colors orange, yellow, and orange-yellow (depending on symptoms) for three days. In this way the integrity of the colon is protected, cleansed and balanced gently, rather than attacked and dried out.

Another difference between traditional naturopathy and Ayurveda, is the primary forms of detoxifying the system. The uses of harsh and system-shocking detoxes are typical in the traditional naturopathic realm. Many of these detoxes are based on organ detoxifying herbs for the kidneys, liver, etc. Many times these detoxes will push the poisons out of an organ into the colon only to be reabsorbed by the blood stream. This is because the colon has not been balanced—the dosha appropriate carriers have not been given. Even massage (abhyanga) is an essential part of the detox in Ayurveda. Massage with the dosha appropriate oils will loosen deep seated toxins in the tissues and help to work them out of the system.

Ayurveda and Chinese medicine both speak of prana and chi or in the case of Orgonomy, orgone, which is the life force. This is what acupuncturists work with and this is what directs your body to elicit a healing response. What if someone has depleted prana/chi and they attempt to detoxify their body? They may be harming their body more than helping. This is because a body that is depleted energetically will become even more depleted, making detox efforts far more debilitating than helpful. We must strive to build up or shall I say "free up" our life force through herbs, yoga, massage, Orgonomy and acupuncture first. It is only after our bodies balance, the elements or the yin/yang--cold and hot--that we will start making our way back towards healing and health.

Some naturopathic therapies recommend an extended period of juicing and raw foods as a means of strengthening or detoxifying the system. While I do not doubt or question the importance of raw living foods on any living organism, I propose the importance of looking at foods in a dosha-specific light using the air/vata example again. Ayurveda says that raw cold juices and vegetables will cause too much dryness and air in the intestines.

The raw food diet will actually cause an air constitution to be excess and in turn, cause constipation and paranoid behavior.

I also question the introduction of carrot juice to the diet. This is often a staple of juicing and is quite high in sugar. Carrot juice will exacerbate any candida infection by actually feeding it. The focus has often become about obsessive trends rather than about sustaining a balanced perspective. This is where I feel Ayurveda has hit the mark. It preserves the integrity of the human body, spirit and soul and gently nudges the body toward health.

Chapter 5

The Aurore Healing Method

A Millennial Advance for Humanity

I wrote this book based on a strong need to "break it all down" for my clients--and for myself. I could spend hours with each person explaining where each theory and treatment derived and could offer numerous examples, both from personal and external experiences. A book was an absolute necessity; a means to bring such complex ideas together into one all-encompassing document. Explaining the method will also supply enough information to let people research all the different treatments for themselves.

To my surprise, in 2008, I sent out my book to be reviewed by a highly respected natural scientist, who also offered a recommendation to study with a psychologist on the west coast. This doctor specialized in orgone therapy and was trained through a colleague of Reich. This recommendation was golden; after flying out to Oregon to meet the doctor, I immediately seized this chance of a lifetime. During this time, I made the pleasant discovery that naturopathy and natural healing are finally being taken more seriously by the medical orgone community. While drugging of patients is sometimes necessary, it is believed that some patients can go farther in their mental health crisis through natural means and should be allowed to do so if possible.

This new change and training has now brought a more complete and thorough aspect to the Aurore method. It is a complex set of treatments aimed at gently waking up the human body's ability to heal. I believe at some point during a person's journey towards health they reach a crisis of belief. Reich affectionately calls this the "kiss of truth." When that happens, one needs to be surrounded by caring individuals who are enlightened and compassionate enough to help them. For some individuals, that crisis of belief will not come because they have comfortably assimilated their illness into their life. This is not a process of coercion by the doctor but of timing, sheer acceptance, love, understanding, and above all, hope.

I felt there was a great need for the this method after many diverse experiences in alternative healing realms, some positive and some not. I give the example that most of us are locked up in a cage, like Hansel in the story of Hansel and Gretel. Some of us can see the key within reach but are too weak or too scared to grab it for ourselves. This is when Gretel comes, to open up the cage, so Hansel can walk out of the cage, willingly, by himself. Many healing methods take the key and leave it within sight but completely out of reach. Others attempt to open the cage and carry the person out. This only increases the chances that the person will fall and revert back into the cage out of fear and uncertainty.

Aspects of the Aurore Method

When I started implementing Ayurveda into my natural healing practice, I felt it was necessary to explore all aspects of the ancient healing science. Many Ayurvedic practitioners in the US ignore essential parts and just focus on the diet, which to me, is not enough. I learned sound and color healing through Ayurveda and also through Dinshah's color light therapy. I also learned about gem recommendations and sidereal astrology, the importance of massage (abhyanga), and the nadi system of acupressure.

I think all of it is relevant. Perhaps there is a general fear that the American public won't accept the entire package, but I don't think that is fair to assume. Just as children move away from baby food and learn to accept what adults eat, many in the holistic community are able to absorb and use more information than has been currently acknowledged. So, part of this method is bringing in all aspects of ayurveda, traditional Chinese medicine, craniosacral therapy, and aspects of Orgonomy.

CranioSacral Therapy and Orgone Therapy

Up until now, CST (CranioSacral therapy) and Orgonomy have been at somewhat opposite ends of alternative therapy. This may be partly because Reich, the founder of Orgonomy, was not focused on the Craniosacral system but his work on muscular armoring is strangely similar to Upledger's somato-emotional release. Perhaps Upledger's discovery of the SomatoEmotional Release *was* spontaneous (Upledger 2002). Upledger merely "stumbled" on to what Reich already knew and had proven 50 years before. Upledger used the term "energy cysts" to describe what Reich had termed "armor" a half a century earlier. I use the word perhaps for Upledger because so many people now are trying to make Reich's work and research their own. The truth is, Reich did the research, Reich sacrificed his life and instead of people rallying behind his work many seek to profit from it themselves and make it their own.

Modern science is constantly "rediscovering" Reich's work and research. This seems unfair because Reich gave his entire life to Orgonomy and even though his work is not been "disproved," the medical community cannot see fit to give credit where credit is due. An example of this is Alexythymia, a term invented by Harvard psychiatrist Peter Sifneos. This is an attempt to describe an apathetic social disease where people cannot find words for their feelings (Levy, 1998). Armoring or "Alexythymia" as Sifneos calls it, was already researched, proven and treated by Reich, again, a half century prior.

There is a serious concern in the Orgonomy community regarding the use of CST for SomatoEmotional release, and for a good reason. The Orgonomist I interviewed said it was because many of these Craniosacral therapists are not qualified as doctors and psychiatrists to handle emotional issues (Applebaum, 2004).

Anyone who has gone through CST knows that emotional releases do happen. An emotionally-releasing CST session can be likened at times to a gentle form of Orgone therapy.

My mother recently shared with me her own encounter with her emotions in a CST session. She was at a resort lying on the beach, seemingly happy and enjoying the sun. She was offered a massage (as part of her package); she followed a man into his massage office and the session commenced. He applied some CST techniques and the next thing she knew she was upset and crying. When the session was over, as she tried to hold in the tears and repress whatever emotions had made their way to the surface, she had to make her way back to the beach.

This is what makes CST so very important. Many of us are not used to being touched and that can make it is quite easy to elicit an emotional response. The Craniosacral therapists are often working within a specific time frame and many do not know how to handle strong emotional responses. Patients can leave the office literally broken in spirit some way or even suicidal if they are not attended to properly. While I believe CST is an important therapy for most people, I also believe there is a middle ground that is worth pursuing.

I utilize CST in the Aurore Healing Method or AHM and I don't use a time frame (typically a session can go from one to three hours). When I get to a restriction in CST, like an occiput (the back of the head) that is stressed and stuck, I hold it and I don't let go. This is important because in CST, when a person is looking for relief, you cannot put a timetable on the body's ability to release emotions. Also, when I see a client starting to go through some emotions, I may hold back and let them experience the treatment over the course of several sessions. I would do this after telling him or her ahead of time what could happen and having qualified professionals available to assist them further.

What has been working best for me is letting the client experience any emotion comes to the surface. I let them enter the flow of that feeling and then supply a bed for the client to hit and kick as much as they feel the need. Then I refer them to an Orgonomist that can work with them in that area, should they choose to do so.

This is a revolutionary approach. Emotional releases are a fact of CST and they can be used for the betterment of the client. Until now, there has been a misunderstood and often downplayed importance on the serious advantages of CST methodology. Some practitioners treat it as simply another "notch in the belt", only to add more initials after their name without fully studying or comprehending the methodology (as with Rolfing now). The truth is, it is much more significant than that.

Americans have clearly reached a point where their bodies are screaming out to release and express themselves. Fifty years ago, life was largely lived according to the status quo. If you were gay, you got married and tried to repress your homosexuality. If you were date raped, you would have to hide your secret for dear life. Hidden pregnancies, hidden loves, hidden problems…but things are starting to change. Now, you see self-expression on a grander scale; it is talked about, openly valued, of greater importance. Many people realize that self-expression is critical and are physically and emotionally sick of hiding their need for it.

Color, Sound, and Flowers: A Match Made in Heaven

Color and sound are important, beneficial tools that I use for healing. In my sessions I choose the correct color for the problem that they present. I usually choose a color for the emotional block for the first few sessions, and then choose another one for the illness in subsequent sessions. As I have mentioned before, color therapy is amazingly effective for physical, emotional and economical reasons.

I have enhanced my timing and expanded the results of using color therapy by adding sound. I use variants of the Pythagorean octave and lower Ayurvedic/yogic tuning forks. The formula I use is simply to take the high frequency of color and divide it by octaves until I get to the closest number for a sound frequency, since sound has a much lower frequency (Dinshah, 2005).

It was during my studies of Dinshah's color therapy when I realized potential flaws within the chakra color system. I propose that when an individual is meditating on the chakras that they visualize in alternate colors that activate and stimulate the chakras. For example, in the chakra system you are told to focus on the color blue for the throat. The color blue is a thyroid-depressing color and the color orange is an activating one for thyroids. In the same way, the pineal and pituitary glands are activated by the color green. The chakra system, however, instructs us to focus the third eye, where the pineal gland is located, on the color purple or indigo. In a country like the United States, many of us suffer from low thyroid and hormonal problems due to environmental exposure, processed food, etc. I feel it is prudent to follow Dinshah's color recommendations, where healing and revitalization is the desired result, rather than the chakric. The Chakric system follows a different non-physical layer of the body and is overly simplified.

I also use flower essence therapy and constitutional homeopathy, both of which I consider as absolutely necessary. I now make my own flower essence called Auror'essence. I find it to be much stronger and more effective than the store-bought variety. It's not that the store-bought variety does not work, but that flower essences are vibrational. This means that their delicate vibrations are effected by where they are kept. Many are packaged and sent on aircraft, sent through magnetic devices, and stored by devices with strong electro-magnetic fields. In my essence, I use crystals, flowers, color, and sound. I keep it within a copper pyramid with a two-inch ruby capstone. Underneath the pyramid, the essence sits atop a copper ayurvedic yantra grid and is surrounded by magnetites and quartz. The pyramid itself was handmade to the exact specification of the Great Pyramid of Giza (Gurudas, 1989).
All of this loving detail makes for a truly comprehensive
and powerful flower essence.

If you have not had good results with flower essences, and this rule also applies to doctors, treatments, therapies, and other methodologies, it is often either the intention to blame for its ineffectiveness, or the actual physical circumstance; i.e, you have good product or idea and it gets ruined by outside circumstances. These can include a good doctor in a cold, ugly office, a good massage therapist with an uncomfortable massage table, and even a good chef in a restaurant filled with a nasty, incompetent wait staff. Many successful endeavors are dependent on outside circumstances. The same applies to wellness: a careful orchestration is needed to bring desired results.

A Promising Hope for Health: Homeopathy

Homeopathic psychology holds amazing possibilities for physical and emotional health. It involves the peeling-away of psycho symptomatic layers to get to a healthier core inner-self. It is based on "constitutional" homeopathy, which is a relatively new trend. It is based on fitting homeopathic remedies to personality profiles and goes so far as to be able to balance such emotional problems as schizophrenia, impulsiveness, insecurity, mania, and any other personality traits or "disorders". I have used it myself to treat all sort of emotional "armors" and defenses that inadvertently and negatively affect health. Rather than changing a person's constitution, it ends up balancing it to a healthier and more habitable form.

    I had a client who exhibited most of the symptoms required for the remedy lycopodium. The person physically suffered from abdominal bloating, hemorrhoids, liver problems and life-long migraines. More than that, the client was always getting sties in the right eye: lycopodium is prone to right-sided complaints. Emotionally speaking, the person expressed a large amount of bravado, which was a mask to cover up deep-seated insecurity. One strange characteristic is that the person does not want to admit that they are sick (lying to prevent others from learning about his or her weakness is another attribute). It helped out immensely that my client was able to admit that, for most people cannot. So, on our first visit, the client left with a recommendation for the remedy lycopodium. I was delighted to find out the weekly sties stopped recurring and the hemorrhoids and bloating stopped as well. However, the migraines were persistent.

This was not the end of my client's journey toward health; after three months of working together, once every two weeks we uncovered several layers of psychosomatic defenses. The person began with lycopodium, which is too right-sided and masculine. After this, the client moved on to anacardium for hypochondria and it is also remedy for people who feel split between different sides of themselves. Some use the term "good and evil" but I don't like to because it moralizes psychological distress. What is really happening is that the person is having a difficult time integrating parts of his or her personality; the side that is too kind and gentle side fights the side that is angry and mean.

Following the anarcardium, I ended my client's treatment with natrum muriaticum. This remedy deals with repressed emotional pain based on conditional love by a parent who was either too smothering or too distant. My client started physically exhibiting symptoms of fluid retention, weight gain, and emotional guilt about a week after we stopped the anarcardium. I could see that the person was covering up emotions and not with the same wall previously with the lycopodium but with a now cold out of touch reticence. I recommended natrum muriaticum, and the results were amazing. After two weeks, the person reported a cloud being lifted. This client also reported, in a six-month follow-up, that the migraines were gone.

I was able to acquire this information, not just by talking about it and having clients fill out a traditional homeopathic case evaluation, but by working with them through craniosacral therapy, color, and sound, and letting them release their feelings. Only after several visits with a client am I finally able to come to homeopathic conclusions, and even then it is usually with some reluctance on the client's part. This is because the further away you get from the physical and the closer you get to the core emotional issue, the more the fight or flight defense of the client become an insurmountable wall to have to bring down.

While I believe whole-heartedly in homeopathy, I have some significant reservations for three important reasons. First of all, in order for homeopathy to work effectively, the person has to avoid coffee and mint. I can get my clients to change toothpastes, but I have an impossible time trying to get them to give up coffee. I have found that even if the say they will, they usually won't and then the remedies become a waste of time and money (coffee does not always antidote the remedies but it could give botched results). Secondly, homeopathy is an exacting science: you have to be 100% on target as to what remedy you need, or otherwise it is a waste of time and money.

The third reason for my discomfort with homeopathy involves the emotional aspects of treating someone with constitutional homeopathy. The process can be quite difficult for both the practitioner and client. A practitioner needs to spend sufficient time with the client in order to access their emotional body. Since most of emotional defenses and armors are below the conscious level, it is difficult to let them know what remedy you are giving them and why.

Typically, people feel defensive. Thus they deliberately and obstinately set up a wall. People are faced with the possibility of walking away from the rain cloud that has been following them around their whole life. In some ways, they love it and hate it. This is what makes constitutional homeopathy so difficult. This is also the reason why self-diagnosing yourself for your own constitution is impractical. You cannot see yourself as clearly as others can. I often think how powerful it would be if more Orgonomists, Rolfers, and Gestalt practitioners employed constitutional homeopathy. Clearly, there is hope to heal, but again, it takes an orchestrated effort.

Please see my references in the appendix for some excellent books and resources on constitutional homeopathy, Rolfing, and Orgonomy.

Perception and Intention: The Cornerstones of Health

Our life on earth is governed by two primary forces: perception and intention. The word *karma* has relevance here. Perception, as I have mentioned in previous chapters, governs how we "see" things and how we process different experiences. It is a primal foundation laid down in the earliest years of life. Trust and security are primary factors in perception. Think of perception as a filter that catches all the information you come in contact with on a daily basis. Some people say you can change perception, but I beg to differ. I believe that perception is a pattern we fall into, often unconscious and steeped in armors and defenses. Hence, our only chance to change our mental and physical existence lies in our ability to become more conscious. Becoming aware of how we perceive things and why we do what we do is liberating, and ultimately, it offers our only chance for emotional freedom. In watching ourselves and understanding why we choose to act the way we do, we change karma-we change the world.

Another, important aspect to healing and life was taught to me by my yoga instructor, Pamela Alexander, whom I have affectionately coined "Kumari." She has taught me over and over that it is not what you do, but how and why you do it. This is the power of intention. I can be excellent and learned at any profession, but the only thing that truly sets me apart from others is my level of intention. Intention is a deciding factor in any outcome, whether I want to help people out of love and compassion, or whether I want to have children out of love and compassion. We can readily see how the power of intention has influenced all parts of our society and affected our ability to be healed and to be well.

The issue of intention takes us right back to Orgonomy and its focus on perception. Many of us believe we are creating seeds of love, when in reality we are sowing seeds of hate. That is, we believe we have good intentions, but our actions do not come across to others that way. I can give an example of this in my own. When going through an impending divorce with my husband, I cried out, "You never loved me." He responded, "Yes, I did, the love was always there, you just didn't see it." Clearly, the message is that we often entertain ourselves by thinking we are lovingly helping, and healing people, but we are not. If others cannot see the love and feel the love, then obviously there is something wrong. Was it my perception or my husband's intentions that caused our marriage to disintegrate? It has to be both.

Too often the breakdown between one human and another is the failure to make authentic contact. The power of underlying negative emotions, which manifest as resentment, can become all encompassing. Yet, by contrast, even as we complain about not getting enough love or not being loved, many of us, when faced with true love and intimacy, run from it and not to it. This is where it is complex, where we have to face the fact that many of us have been unwilling to make a choice. We have spouses that cannot love us and spouses we cannot love. Instead of resolving or focusing to mend these issues, we spend our time continually complaining about them for the rest of our lives. In any relationship, one must look at the self first.

People stuck in the role of self-denial who habitually deceive themselves will be nearly impossible to reach. They could be stuck in this mental muddle for the rest of their lives. This is the state of mind where bad is good, good is bad—a state dominated by sarcasm, confusion, and sickness. People continue to lie to themselves, and this is where they can lose their mind and then their health. This is also the place where people lose their spouse, and this is where they lose their children. This is where they desperately need to become conscious and bring awareness into their own lives, all things are possible.

AMH and Bio-therapeutic Yoga are stepping stones to health by simply teaching others to start listening to and trusting themselves. I concentrate first on initiating a healing response from the individual. If I can get them to agree to accept wellness on more than just a superficial level, they then have a greater ability to be healed, to be well, and to be happy. They can thus honor their feelings and know who they are; this in and of itself is a major contribution to the realm of alternative healing, bridging the gap between body and mind, sickness and healing-through acceptance and release.

What is an Aurore Session like?

I try to get each of my clients to come at least four to six times. I consider my first treatment paramount as I have to elicit enough healing responses in the emotional body to get the client to reach the point where they really want to be healed. They have to initially gather enough personal stamina and power to be able to come back for subsequent visits, to take whatever herbs I recommend and to do whatever physical exercises are advised. My client has to understand that I use a multi-dimensional healing formula that encompasses the whole body. Too often I have witnessed friends leave visits to natural doctors with hundreds of dollars in herbs, only to stop taking them within a few days and then to finally dismiss the herbs and treatment and declare that they do not work. This is an obstacle to healing that must be addressed in the first session.

Before my first session I have clients fill out an Ayurvedic symptom inventory. This is so that the client and I can get the most out of our session together. This benefits the client so that when we meet they feel they are truly "getting" something for their money. After I look over the information, I try to come up with a figure in my head as to how psychosomatic their illness is and what area of the body is holding the most illness. This allows me to refer them out to someone else if I have reached my own limits in healing methods.

My sessions run from a half-hour for an Ayurvedic diet consultation all the way up to three hours for the process of initiating stronger healing responses to begin detoxifying the system. The Aurore Method includes but is not limited to; Auror'essence, vita-flex reflexology based on Stanley Burrow's research (Burrows,

1993), color, sound, detox, and craniosacral therapy. The combination of these therapies creates a powerful push in the healing processes of both body and mind. I only attempt to guide and teach my clients to the ultimate truth, which is essentially they, themselves are the healer. Once, they know who they are and how they feel, they begin developing the necessary tools to facilitate self-help and self-diagnosis. Even then, we must continually check ourselves and each other as we journey toward truth and enlightenment.

Conditioned negative responses will never be fully discarded. Accordingly, the real hope is to become actively conscious. Once we become conscious of why and how we do what we do, we can catch ourselves. The problem then becomes working out negative feelings in a proper manner, not repressing them as before. Realizing symptoms of anger and letting go of the guilt associated with expressing them is powerfully freeing. The behavior and feelings that we have can now become a conscious signal that requires a response.

The Goddess Response

For those familiar with Hindu mythology I give examples of the many aspects of the Goddess Devi to help highlight this particular response. This Goddess can manifest herself as Parvati, the wife of Shiva and mother of Ganesha, a symbol of nourishing love and unconditional acceptance. She is portrayed delicately usually on a lotus flower. She can also become durga, which is the Goddess of protection and strength. Durga has many arms carrying weapons and rides a tiger. When the Goddess is pushed and no other outlet can be found, she becomes the deadly Goddess, Kali. Kali wears a necklace of human skulls and she symbolizes death, destruction and hatred. When the rage of Kali is awakened things happen that are not easily reversed or turned back. Many of us strive to live like the loving Goddess Parvati (for Christian's, this is Mother Mary or aspects of Jesus), but we are actually manifesting inward and outwardly the aspects of Kali in an unhealthy way. We store and deny our anger and rage until we explode on an unsuspecting object or person in our path, causing irreversible damage and quite often serious regret and guilt.

If we can become more like Durga, who is both loving and protective, we balance the anger and hatred of Kali (that lives in us all) and also the divine love of Parvati (which also lives in us all). The key then is to put away self-loathing and replace it with the balanced perspective of acceptance. Acceptance is always the most tangible and necessary aspect of divine love. Without acceptance there is no love.

Aurore Yoga: Peace through Release

I came up with the idea to create an orgone centered biotherapeutic Yoga during my Orgonomy treatments. I always knew that yoga and meditation were powerful tools to calm and strengthen the body and promote greater conscious awareness. I also knew that yoga and meditation had the ability to take people away from the here and now and keep them from acknowledging their true feelings. I felt like I needed to help create a bridge between all of the benefits of yoga and the benefit of being emotionally honest, with the ability to release energy.

My form of yoga is for the people who are not content with their current yoga practice. If you are practicing yoga and meditation and you are emotionally beating yourself up with guilt for occasional bouts of anger and rage, then you are a good candidate for my Yoga. If you are seeking to create that emotional bliss that you envision yogis and other people you highly esteem have and you cannot do it, then Aurore is for you. If you find yourself meditating, reading self-help books, or perpetually doing things that keep you from dealing with your life circumstances, then Aurore yoga is for you.

In this yoga, I use the basic precepts of traditional yoga asanas, but I include the use of deep open mouth breaths with facial expression. I also take an orgonomic approach and work backwards down the chakras, starting with the head and ending with the pelvis in each session. These may seem like small differences but

The Aurore Method

I assure you they are not. Facial expressions are a very important link between body and mind and it is often suppressed or treated too lightly in yoga classes. The lion pose that is usually done at the end of class is the most important although often the most unappreciated. Everyone is looking around and giggling or simply not doing it, out of fear of "looking stupid". Lion pose activates body and mind and brings deep emotion out into the face. You produce a loud bellowing sound and stick out your tongue and cross your eyes or roll your eyes.

The inhibition behind lion pose is that many of us were spanked when we made faces as a child. Many of us were shamed or told not to make faces because they were not nice. Face making is a part of the soul trying to express itself. Lion pose brings many aspects of the emotional and physical body together and should not be overlooked. The nice thing about the DVD is that you can make all the faces you want and no one is there to laugh at you.

Another aspect of Aurore Yoga is hitting and punching in the yoga session. This seems to be opposite of what yoga is supposed to be about, but it is not if you view yoga as a means toward healing and release. This is perhaps a reason why Budukon™ has caught on so popularly. The general public likes kickboxing or the idea of getting the aggression out in an acceptable, even competitive or constructive manner. Aurore Yoga differs from Budukon™ in the way it handles aggression through intentional hitting, not just hitting to hit. This is unique for yoga but not for Orgonomy. The importance lies in releasing the buried resentment we hold towards others to experience the maximum benefit. First, however, we have to know what we feel. Why we feel it will come secondary because it doesn't necessarily have to make sense us.

Kicking and hitting in a random nonspecific manner, lets you expand energy but the emotional aspects of the resentment have been ignored. In this way your expansion is only superficial and short-lived.

The Emotional Release of Yoga

In various styles of yogic body positions, you may experience a spontaneous emotion coming to the surface. This surface emotion could come in the form of a simple fleeting feeling of anxiety, or a racing heartbeat. It could also be as complex as feeling terror and fear and realization that you are alone. When you reach this point you simply lie down and breathe deeply and ask yourself who it is that made you scared, or made you feel alone. Delve deeper into the spontaneous reflection brought to your attention. Remember, this is about perception and the reasons and excuses are not important. For instance, when I was doing vinyasa yoga a few years ago I was lying down on my stomach with my arms crossed underneath me. We held this pose for a few minutes but it seemed like an eternity. All of a sudden I felt a panic and had the feeling I was being tied up or held down. During corpse pose at the end of class, a memory of my father holding me down when I was little came to mind. He would hold me down and tickle me until my laughing turned to tears and then finally to terror and pain. This type of tickle torture gave him much pleasure and whatever his intentions were, that was not significant to me at the time the memory had floated to the surface. I learned from Orgonomy to let go of the guilt regarding a situation and not to give anyone excuses for bad behavior.

    I went home after my yoga class and kicked and punched on my punching bag for over a half hour. During that time I thought about my dad and the situation. I screamed in a deep voice, "let me go, leave me alone, I hate you, you f------- idiot!" The screaming part never came easy to me and took treatment with my Orgonomist in order to feel comfortable screaming to my parents out loud. The fear of retribution and rejection from my parents was still there, even though I was punching an inanimate object. When I get angry I have to swear; it is my first defense. Perhaps, it is because those words were so bad and forbidden. Also, as a woman, I have grown up knowing that certain

The Aurore Method

words make women "look" bad and are off limits. Whatever it is, I need to do it and when I do I feel better.

Hitting has saved me from lashing out at my husband and children. Another scenario I can offer is that when those feelings came up in my class, I could have felt guilty and stifled them. Then I would have gone home and within a few days got into an argument with my husband. I could have severely damaged my relationship with him (as I have before) by taking my anger out on him. I could have called him the f------- idiot and it would have had nothing (or little) to do with him. Hence, the reason for Aurore Yoga--I believe the world is ready to release.

In my yoga, besides the open mouth breathing and facial expressions, I use the corpse pose as a time to explore feelings. Kicking and punching is employed intermittently throughout yoga, but it is especially important afterwards, especially if during the course of the yoga session, something relevant comes up. Keep in mind it does not happen every session and might take some time for you to "feel" your feelings. The point is to get to know your feelings and when they surface and then immediately undertake the task of getting them out of your body physically. You need the active stretching of yoga and the stillness of corpse pose to gently awaken and release inner feelings. If there is an inclination to cry, by all means do so but do not confuse sadness with anger, as we often do. Often, for women, crying is an acceptable subjugation for anger. For men, cynicism or anger is used to subjugate emotions like fear or sadness to thwart the necessity of crying. Instead of letting out the rage or sadness, we sometimes attempt to diffuse the feelings or change them. The point I am trying to make is, let there be a time, at least once a week, where all aspects of human emotion are welcomed and released.

This variation on traditional yoga presents a revolutionary approach to health and the human body. People who have already gone through Orgonomy treatments will understand the basis fully and it will benefit them between treatments (many people have to travel great distances to see their Orgonomists). For others who have reached the point in their health and fitness where they are ready to take it to the next level, this will be the welcomed next step you've been searching for. We are currently working on a DVD in the near future to guide you and teach you in your home practice. As always, you are never alone and effective help is only a call away, should something strongly emotional come up.

We can say that the human body already has vast amounts of energy stored and compartmentalized in the body. Much of this energy is locked in self-imposed compartments and is unable to flow freely. Aurore Yoga provides a means to gently release pent up energy and allow for access to more energy. Here is a list comparing Aurore to typical yoga practice:

Aurore Yoga:

- Focuses on becoming more aware of the human body and emotions
- Grounding: encourages the ability of the individual to "Be Here Now" and present within the moment, instead of escaping
- Allows for truth and sincerity of all emotions
- Works backwards down the Chakras, the head down
- Deep Mouth Orgone Breathing, instead of nose breathing
- Energy building Pranayama with Orgone breaths between yogic sets
- Kicking, hitting and punching before, during or after yoga.
- Chakras colors based on Dinshah's color therapy.

Chapter Six

Healing Children Simply With Color, Sound and Sleep

I am a homeschooling parent. This means that being a parent is the number one most important job that I have. As you can imagine, it is a tremendous undertaking but I am a firm believer in practicing what I preach. In this way I strive to give my children a natural homeschooling environment with no fluorescent lighting in the home, and no harmful pesticides, fungicides and germicides. As a Mother, Doctor of Natural Health, and home school teacher I believe in the importance of giving children a healthy start and I try my hardest to do what I can, when I can. I make a conscious effort to keep my priorities in check whenever possible. I figure, that since I gave them a natural birth, it is only fitting that I provide them with a natural education as well.

The most important causes of health disturbances in childhood are often overlooked in favor of early and aggressive education. Simple things like sleep deprivation, TV watching, video game playing, lack of access to healthy foods and exposures to toxins and pesticides can create lifelong stumbling blocks to mental and physical health and literal metabolic imbalances. It is sometimes difficult for parents to explore these simple truths. Parents are often looking for a grandfather or uncle to blame that wasn't "quite right" or had some mental issues and disturbances. They typically are not thrilled to hear: turn off the TV and put your child to bed.

I cannot count how many times people have come to me for problems with their children, seeking help only when there is an academic decline or the child isn't meeting the parents intellectual goals. Many times however, I stop parents in their tracks by asking quite simply: how much sleep does your child get a night? How much TV does your child watch? More often then not I get a defensive, reluctant admission that the child is indeed overly scheduled, burned out, and exhausted from school and activities. More often than not, that child is also at the same time being babysat by an electrical box that talks.

I realize that my opinion against TV and video games doesn't hold a lot of water as compared to the benefits that parents get: such as free time to think, work, talk on the phone. Those are true benefits and should not be devalued or over looked. However, if you allow your child to learn how to play and entertain themselves- creatively, those benefits of momentarily escapes are still evident. Another way to convince you is to look at an important law on TV passed in 2008 in France.

TV Outlawed in France

In August 2008, France took a controversial step in banning TV for young children and babies. The French have scientifically proven that TV watching disrupts the brain, slows language and learning. This is no surprise to us Waldorfers (see below) as this is something that has been known and promoted by Steiner organizations for over 70 years but up until now there was no concrete scientific research. The ruling has won the praise of the CCFC or Campaign for Commercial Free Childhood. This is an organization of healthcare professionals and concerned parents who are seeking to protect children from being constantly inundated with commercialism and hypnotic sales tactics. I encourage you to join them if you haven't already; information about it is enclosed below my article here. Dr. Susan Linn from the CCFC says the TV ban "sends a strong message that the health and well-being of children is more important than a businesses bottom line" (Golin, 2008).

Scientific Proof and More...

This proves that when it comes to language learning and coinciding, the need for love and human interaction that it cannot be replaced by a mechanical talking box that gives off strong electromagnetic waves. As a mother of three children that are quad lingual, I really encourage others to bring the gift of language to the child in a way that is contactfully alive. This should come ideally through themselves and not someone else and certainly not through a computer or TV. What is the problem with banning TV from children? Well, why I don't list some of the benefits instead: children forced to play now and hence, act like children, children learning to create and imagine games, art, and toys on their own, children moving more and becoming more active (to the dismay of parents)...the list could go on and on. So, the biggest change is going to need to come from parents and how does one change that? Clearly the first and most important lesson must be tolerance for childhood behavior.

The Bottom Line is Money

It has been my experience that the TV used as an educator/babysitter for an hour is far if not completely inferior to a few minutes of quality human interaction with a child. To quote Kahlil Gibran from The Prophet: "They [the children] come through you but not from you...you may strive to be like them, but seek not to make them like you...You are the bows from which your children as living arrows are sent forth..." Let us not forget, in the hurry to shoot our children out into the world often at times prematurely and irreverently, the time it takes to place the arrow on the quiver to sight it in, to direct it, and pull it back. While, it is easy to put our kids in front of the TV and forget about them and even think we are doing them a favor, but lets not forget the hard part of parenthood which calls us to take the time, reach out, and connect with our kids and give our children something that may have not been given to us. If we continue on in the same path that our own parents had led us down then we in fact causing the future to go backwards and make it like the past, and therefore seeking to make our children like us.

Making a Difference in the Future of Tomorrow

In quoting from The Prophet again: "Their souls dwell in the house of tomorrow....life goes not backwards nor tarries with yesterday." So I encourage all of you, who no doubt care about your children very much, to *never forget* the power you have as a parent to impact your children's lives and how much they will appreciate that gift from you. Similarly, be more confident in your parenting; trust yourself and your own educational abilities. We have been led to believe that only schools can teach but the school of the parent's heart is the first and primary educator. This is not at all meant to imply that there should be no TV watching at all, but to imply the need for age and time appropriate boundaries.

This is one reason why I myself utilize the Waldorf method of teaching at home. The Waldorf method is primarily based on protecting the realm of childhood and giving children ample time to play and be children with rhythm and reverence and not compulsory aggression. Another aspect of the Waldorf method is using (and making) only natural toys, clothes and school supplies. Up until the year 2008 when kids and pets started dying from plastics and poisons in paints from China, I was looked at strangely by many friends and family. People thought I was depriving my children of fun by only giving them natural wood toys. However, after the plastic crisis hit I got many phone calls and apologies, even from my own mother!

This is one reason why I myself utilize the Waldorf method of teaching at home. The Waldorf method is primarily based on protecting the realm of childhood and giving children ample time to play and be children with rhythm and reverence and not compulsory aggression. Another aspect of the Waldorf method is using (and making) only natural toys, clothes and school supplies. Up until the year 2008 when kids and pets started dying from plastics and poisons in paints from China, I was looked at strangely by many friends and family. People thought I was depriving my children of fun by only giving them natural wood toys. However, after the plastic crisis hit I got many phone calls and apologies, even from my own mother!

My change from plastic to no plastic did not happen overnight, but through a gradual realization that it was a hypocritical part of my life that needed to be changed. I was continually frustrated over it and I finally gathered the strength to go more natural then before. Granted that I am typing this on a plastic keyboard! I realize the importance of balance in this area and not obsessive compulsive force.

Health Benefits from Sound and Color

I have researched the health benefits of music, language, color, and sound and have faithfully used it with my own family and practice for the last 12 years. As I mentioned before, color and sound therapy were a very important part of my son's healing from autism. Because color and sound are such an important foundation in the therapies I employ for natural health, I also spend a tremendous amount of time educating others about the uses and benefits of color and sound therapies. In a time of economic uncertainty, color and sound are powerfully effective and economically advantageous means of treatment. With this comes the truth that dependence and addiction to expensive herbal supplements and vitamins are thankfully avoided.

Besides working with parents and children in my office I have also created a DVD and lesson program for parents to do at home with their children. Having its basis in the fore mentioned color and sound therapies it also incorporates aspects Waldorf music education. I have now created a refreshingly different and amazingly effective music and sound therapy program that encompasses all of the arts. In this method the children are learning basic musical principals through the healing aspects of color, sound and language all at the same time.

In terms of music as a form of therapy and lessons, I encourage parents that they can unequivocally have both. There are, of course, lots of classes to expose your child to "music" however, the most important and overlooked aspect of early music learning is the exposure of "pure tones." This is where sound therapy comes in and applying pure tones to the body to balance and bring wellness as in Jean Beaulieu's research on the Pythagorean scale and the interesting work of composer John Cage (Beaulieu, 1995). My music therapy program the AMHC strives to bring sound and color therapy together in a harmonious and fluid intellectual transition.

The colors applied to my song books are not applied half-hazardly for visual appeal but are based on scientific research of color and sound as recommended by Dr. Darius Dinshah, whom I have previously mentioned.

Add a Dash of Music and Foreign Language...

The area of foreign language learning is as diverse as the area of music learning, especially when it comes to early childhood. Everyone seems to know the "earlier the better" research but many feel lost and confused as to how to approach these two important subjects. Brain scans have now proven that the bridge between the two sides of the brain, the corpus callosum, is actually 15 percent larger in adults who started music lessons before the age of eight than in those who started later. The corpus callosum carries a hundred million nerve fibers; a 15% increase in its cross-section suggests a vast increase in information flow (Jourdain, 2002). Similar research has been recorded about children who grew up bilingually with an increase in the density of gray brain matter (Hitti, 2008). An early experience with music and foreign language has a profound effect on the performance of the brain and the entire human body.

The fact that the majority of American music education is spent on learning music, rather than creating it, shows that music learning is not a perfect science and could be dramatically improved upon (Jourdain). Another sad but true fact is that foreign language is not routinely taught until after the ages of 12 to 14 years old in the United States. This compelling research has not caught up to or yet changed an educational system that holds on to out dated concepts and that has, in many ways, failed our children in the area of the Arts.

So, do we as parents aggressively over intellectualize our children, to get all of their "early" training in with grand hopes of virtuosity and genius mentality? Indeed, not, I propose that a child's intellect can be both trained musically and protected reverently. One way we can accomplish task is to first ask ourselves what our ultimate motives and goals are for our child. This question should help us first, create an age appropriate lesson structure which honors the child and secondly, to help the child develop a life long appreciation of music and language.

Memorization vs. Comprehension

I will never forget the wise words spoken by my children's former music teacher on the last day of my seven year olds class. She said, "Resist the temptation to have them perform and memorize songs at the expense of slowly building solid technique and understanding." Her words illuminated in my mind as I recently re-read the book "The Miracle Worker" the story of Helen Keller, a child that was deaf and blind and her relationship with her teacher Anne Sullivan. While, Helen's parents were more than satisfied and truly impressed to have their daughter perform memorized signs and imitate proper behavior for treats, Ms. Sullivan was not. Ms. Sullivan would not rest or give up until Helen understood what the signs meant and developed "comprehension." This comprehension was only made possible by forming a relationship with the child, remaining steadfast, and finally by the child opening her heart on her own accord and began to "trust" the teacher.

This story is microcosmically related because every parent strives to balance the polarized aspects of Helen's mother and Anne

Sullivan throughout parenthood. In my work with autistic children, healing is often only possible when the Helen's Mother *within the parent voluntarily* surrenders and the Ann Sullivan within the parent takes command. Macrocosmically speaking, I cannot help but question how many Helen Keller's have the traditional educational system produced? How many children are playing music, to play, with memorization and lack of comprehension? How many children speak words without meaning? Have teachers that haven't taught? Or parent's that have simply given up?

To answer my musical education questions, I turn to Brian DiBlassio, an assistant Professor of music at the University of Michigan. Besides his university work, Mr. DiBlassio also maintains a base of private teaching for children. He says that teachers can often be afraid to let the natural, creative, ear-based playing run wild because they don't know how to embrace and develop it. They can often be more comfortable with tangible, traditional skills that are easier to quantify (curl your fingers, that is a middle C, etc.). He also remarked that his own love and development for music came directly from his mother, who introduced him at nine years old but never made it compulsory or abusive. This "gentle" introduction to music has given him the freedom to both follow music into a successful career and continue to find residual joy in creating music, day after day and year after year.

Mr. DiBlassio had a very specific and enlightening response when asked about music learning. I found it so profound and courageously intriguing; I decided to quote him directly and keep it in its entirety. "I think there is an *extremely* delicate balance in how one should unfold the art of playing and communicating music while teaching children. Starting the child off too early with note reading, the logic of counting, and intense hand techniques will risk overload and increase a later propensity to music repulsion. Teaching the child totally by ear, too far in their intellectual development, could potentially cause an enormous deficit of musical reading and writing that takes years of focus and commitment to overcome.

Surprisingly, I believe the musician who learns completely by ear and can't read a note can be just as musical or MORE musical than one who learns both skills. However, this completely ear-based musician will have a quite difficult, if not impossible time functioning and communicating as a musician in society (exactly analogous to a brilliant adult who can't read or write).

Specifically, I believe children from womb to about 7 years should have music in their environment -- daily. Actively listening, singing/being sung to, freedom to play a variety of instruments in the household. If they begin an instrument in this time period, it should be offered with no expectations, like a meal set before them. If they are hungry fine, if not, back off!

Age 8 to . . . 24(?) would be a good time to offer more formal lessons that combine the intellectual skills of technique and theory with the listening and playing artistry of music.

From age 18(?) to ___ would be a good time to talk about using music as a form of meditation with the possibilities of transcending consciousness."

Musicality, Mental Illness and More

I can't tell you the sigh of relief I had after reading Professor DiBlassio's response to music learning. It changed my sometimes biased views and assumptions of the educational system. It made me realize that the educational system, just like any system or group, is absolutely diverse and capable of progress and change. But what about the term musicality, or the ability to be musical, sometimes described as having an "ear" for music? It is strongly dependent on the first years of life. The musical sphere can be strongly influenced by neurosis and Reich proved all primary neurosis is cemented within the first four years of life (Reich, 1972).

Besides research I cited earlier about ultrasound damaging the ear drums, thus producing tone deafness, there is also a psychological aspect of music learning which is strong influenced by the mother and child relationship. In Reich's book "Character

Analysis" he described a neurotic male's lack of coordination, muscular armoring and resistance to music as being traced to his first years of life. This man had an emotionally rejecting and contactless relationship with his mother that made him libidinally frustrated and thus produced longing and muscular tension within his body. The man's mother attempted to sustain the relationship with her son through singing, perhaps out of a replacement for attachment that she was either consciously or unconsciously aware of.

The child picked up on his mother's attempt to sublimate relationship through music and instead of being comforted by his mother's voice he became more aware of his "love" disappointment. His initial excitement for music made him muscularly tense because of the emotions brought to the surface which were innately connected to his unrewarding relationship with his mother. These feelings produced a vegetative excitation because of his inability to gratify his instinctual impulses. Thus, the feelings brought to the surface through listening to music were then held tightly in the body through repression and then subsequently experienced as anxiety. The anxiety attacks continued on for this man into adulthood until he finally got help through Orgone therapy.

So, the immense pleasure that music can bring to the human body is subjective to early childhood experiences. Music can be a helpful emotional trigger producing healing if the person is aware of their character resistance. However, music can also become a detrimental player in character reaction formations which produce emotional stasis, anxiety and mental illness. This research serves as a reminder to all parents to protect the not only the parent child relationship, but also the musical sphere. Resisting the urge to harm the child musically through mechanical neurotic impulses may prove to be a strong factor in producing a healthy adult musician, if in fact that is one's goal.

More on Foreign Language

Since my children were born I have not only exposed them to pure tones and sound therapy but I have taught them French, German, and Spanish along with English. This seemed to be a waste of time for my son who was autistic, as he ignored all my jibber jabber. However, his memory served him well because when his autism subsided all the years of foreign language and pure tone exposure dramatically surfaced. He has now perfect pitch and this was a child that I thought one time was deaf! Foreign language develops an expanded thinking capacity and develops the brain. I ignored early educational models of early reading and writing in favor of music, art and foreign language exposure.

For foreign language introduction, many parents are relying solely, if not completely on tapes and DVD, but what about the research that shows TV before 7 years old can be very damaging (2004)? Children under seven thrive, need and learn through real interaction especially with music, rhymes, singing and signing. (Why signing? I use English Sign Language as a "base" physical language to link all other languages). At one point on my language journey with my own children, I enrolled them in L'Ecole de Francaise, a French immersion school for expatriates. There they got the much needed immersion but were unfortunately surrounded by teachers who were so cruel to them they did not want to speak French anymore! Thus, after the plan having backfired, I had to seek out a better solution that left me, the parent in ultimate control.

Let me make it clear, I pass no judgment on parents resorting to TV for language immersion because I understand the parents' plight. As a parent and an early music and language educator I have struggled with this and still do. My older two children had many hours of diverse language TV time, programs like: Muzzy, Lyric Language, TinTin, etc. None of these videos, however, helped to produce the language savvy individuals I had hoped for and any language learning they learned came directly from me and my not so desirable accent! Similarly, in the musical realm the long distance traveling to the very expensive Kelly Kirby piano classes at five years old proved to be little more than overwhelming my children with "adult-erated" expectations at the expense of their childhood. I speak of childhood as a sacred realm, an area that needs to be tread upon with great care and appreciation.

About the Program

The AMHC Phase I is the first in a series of three programs. It contains charming folk songs in French, German, and Spanish led by children; indeed, the songbook itself was designed and created with the help of children. Created in a pentatonic octave, there is no annoying dissonance. This means that children are introduced to sound and music foundation with great confidence and compositional abilities. The lesson planner is filled with ideas and lessons for children of all ages and adults. The DVD that comes with the program isn't meant for children to sit and watch over and over although they will want to but as a means to inspire and help with pronunciation. Along with a translation guide and a pronunciation guide in the song book, you have a complete educational program which is simple and easy to comprehend.

I encourage anyone interested in early childhood education to thoughtfully consider using temperance and careful evaluation, even considering health and psychology, when forming goals and expectations for their child. I leave you with a quote to inspire you on your journey from the founder of Waldorf schools, Rudolf Steiner, "Receive children in reverence, educate them in love, and send them forth in freedom."

Chapter 7

Naturopathic Psychotherapy, the Time has Come

This is the most important chapter in the book. This subject is very controversial and one not lightly treaded upon. Still, it presents the urgent issue—one that screams out for all of us to listen to.

Up until now I have made some basic references to psychosomatic illness and how anger and emotions are held in the body. But on a more specific level, my work as a doctor of natural health has led me to repeated encounters with mental disease. Whether we want to deal with it or "not" in one form or the other, it is a pervasive problem and affects far too many to be ignored or glossed over. Many people I see are confessing a natural lifestyle and yet, to their dismay and sometimes shame, they are drugging themselves or one of their loved ones to help control the symptoms of mental distress.

I know what kind of strong reaction this kind of information invokes so before we start this chapter I would like to set some parameters:

First of all, there are some mental illnesses which are undoubtedly severe, including catatonic schizophrenia, mania, and the condition of being an unfeeling sociopath, just to name a few. I exercise caution in this area and only the individual reading this knows whether they or the person they love are "that" far gone and to what degree. Similarly, I already mentioned that I am in no way in favor of all American's getting off the meds and this is indeed the area for only licensed psychologists.

What I am going to discuss is the possibility that many who are drugging themselves for mental instability may actually be able to function without drugs and work towards healing and mental stability. The most recent statistics on mental health drugs use such as psychotropics in the United States is truly jaw dropping. As of May 5, 2009, 73 percent more adults and 50 percent more children are using drugs to treat mental illness than in 1996 (Steenhuysen, 2009). Well, you maybe wondering what were the numbers in 1996 and so am I. The article carefully neglected to mention those numbers so I had to research them myself. I found that the U.S. Centers for Disease Control and Prevention reported 2.4 billion drugs prescriptions in 2005. Of those, 118 million were for antidepressants.

The article went on to say that the new jump in mental illness drug prescriptions are attributed to recent expaned pharmaceutical drug coverage and the new found ease in the ability of primary care physicians to diagnose mental illness and prescribe to adults and children. We should not be surprised at the information that the drug companies stand to gain immensely with 200 million people (or more) on antidepressants. While this staggering information appears dark and hopeless, there is a light in the tunnel. There are medical doctors out there that are truly working to protect their patients' best interests.

For this, I quote an article about antidepressants and a doctor who chooses not to be sold out to drug companies. "Dr. Robert Goodman, an internist in New York City, says the real force behind skyrocketing antidepressant prescription rates is pharmaceutical marketing to doctors and to consumers." You put those two together and you get a lot of prescriptions for antidepressants," he said. He questions whether all those prescriptions are necessary. "It's hard to believe that number of people is depressed, or that antidepressants are the answer," he said. Goodman is the founder of a group called "No Free Lunch," a group that encourages doctors to reject gifts from pharmaceutical companies. He added that patients sometimes see ads for antidepressants on television and ask doctors for the drugs -- and that studies show these requests work (Cohen, 2007).

Happy Pills, Are You Serious?

Time and time again I have heard anti-depressants or more specifically SSRIs referred to as "happy pills." Maybe you are wondering what the big deal is about taking a little happy pill as long as the government gives the thumbs up. Here is a partial list of SSRIs taken from the informative website about the dangerous side effects of SSRIs called www.ssristories.com. Please keep in mind that pharmaceuticals are constantly changing their names all the time. Selective Serotonin Reuptake Inhibitors (SSRIs), of which Prozac was the first. Other SSRIs are Zoloft, Paxil (Seroxat), Celexa, Sarafem (Prozac in a pink pill), Lexapro, and Luvox. Other newer antidepressants included in this list are Remeron, Anafranil and the SNRIs Effexor, Serzone and Cymbalta as well as the dopamine reuptake inhibitor antidepressant Wellbutrin (also marketed as Zyban).

The SSRI story website also lists 3,000 news stories mainly *criminal* in nature that have appeared in the media or were part of FDA testimony in 1991, 2004 or 2006, in which antidepressants are mentioned. Did the word "criminal" get your attention? Well it should, there are over 48 school shootings, over 600 murders (homicides), over 180 murder- suicides connected to SSRI use listed on the site.

Have noticed an increase of entire family murders within the last year? We have been told by the media that it is caused from the economic downturn. What you won't find easily in the press is what "legal" medication the people involved in the incident were taking. Seldom, have I myself personally, read in any of these accounts that the person had lost their job or suffered a type of economic financial crisis (of course, we are all from time to time in the midst of these crisis). Yet, we are told that the "economy" did it. This is now reminding me of the vaccine cover up story I had mentioned earlier.

As if being on the SSRI's and having or experiencing more mental illness than before isn't enough, apparently withdrawal from the drugs is worse than being on them. Again to quote the

SSRI website they list an FDA list about the apparent dangers of the drugs.

FDA Public Health Advisory

On March 22, 2004 the FDA published a Public Health Advisory that reiterates several side effects and states (in part) "Anxiety, agitation, panic attacks, insomnia, irritability, hostility, impulsivity, akathisia (severe restlessness), hypomania, and mania have been reported in adult and pediatric patients being treated with antidepressants for major depressive disorder as well as for other indications, both psychiatric and non-psychiatric."

1. On September 14, 2004 the FDA added a Black Box Warning in regard to antidepressants & suicidality in those under age 18.

2. On September 14, 2004 the FDA mandated that pharmacies provide to all parents or guardians for those younger than 18 an *Antidepressant Patient Medication Guide*. This guide reads (in part) "Call healthcare provider right away if you or your family member has any of the following symptoms: Acting aggressive, being angry, or violent & acting on dangerous impulses." This *Antidepressant Patient Medication Guide* also states "Never stop an antidepressant medicine without first talking to a healthcare provider. Stopping an antidepressant medicine suddenly can cause other symptoms."

3. On December 13, 2006, the Black Box Warning for suicidality was updated to include those under age 25. The Black Box Warning is included in the insert to the drugs and in the Physicians' Desk reference.

SSRIs Tragedies Becoming More Frequent

Early in 2009 a friend of mine through my homeschool group was viciously murdered in a family murder-suicide, her name was Francie Billotti-Wood. Francie was a natural living activist; she was helpful, full of life, married and had three beautiful children. I was shocked to find out one morning on the news that she and her three sweet children were murdered by her husband. It didn't make sense to me, although I never met him and only knew her through the web group and our correspondences, the situation did not add up.

Francie was the more serious one in the relationship and from what I knew about her husband, Chris, he was the funny and easy-going one. She was obsessed with healthy living and was meticulous about her regimen. He appeared for the most part to graciously go along. Although she never told me personally, I found out through her blog that she started taking antidepressants after the birth of her third child. Knowing Francie, this must have been a difficult decision for her to make but she did have three small children under five and was desperately trying to cope. Her blog was strangely entitled "What am I supposed to do now?" as if she was revealing her anxiety and frustration with her home life.

I found Francie's behavior to become more erratic within the last year, which maybe explained by the SSRI use. She had just moved to Maryland from Florida and within a month or two she was obsessing about moving again. At that time, I imagined that this behavior was causing a stress on the marriage and family. But all of that seemed meaningless after her husband's savage and psychotic murder spree of mental illness, which shocked me to the core. Not only did he shoot them but he also nearly decapitated them.

Was her husband Chris also using SSRI's? I never knew until after they died. Officials seized four different types of antidepressants that he had been prescribed (Galucci-White, 2009). They were were: Cymbalta (duloxetine), alprazolam (a benzodiazepine) paroxetine (Paxil), and buspirone (BuSpar)]. BuSpar is an anti-anxiety drug which, unlike the anti-anxiety benzodiazepines, raises serotonin levels in the brain.

Who Killed 4-Year-Old Rebecca Riley?

The age for diagnosing mental illness is rapidly decreasing to appease the outcry of parents that are searching for ways to deal with childhood. Again, I go back to my previous quote on Reich about the misery of an infant in the hands of armored parents, clearly this is the case here. A few years ago it was thought that schizophrenia could not be diagnosed until 18 years of age, now you have children as young as two years old being diagnosed and treated with psychotic drugs and SSRIs. Take for example the tragic and needless death of 4 year old Rebecca Riley who was diagnosed with ADD and bi- polar disease at 2 ½ years old. She was drugged and drugged by her parents and family doctor until she died (Raja, 2007).

The coroner found lethal doses of Clonidine (to stabilize her moods), Seroqel (anti-psychotic), Depakote (for bi-polar), an anti-histamine, and a cough suppressant in her blood. During the day the parents told her to take her "happy medicine" and at night the parents gave her extra which they coined the "sleepy medicine." The school that Rebecca attended, when interviewed after her death, said that she would arrive at school floppy, weak, and shaking badly. Neighbors described all of the Reilly children as "little robots" (La Voie, 2007).

In a more thorough investigation of Rebecca's family it was found that the father, Michael Riley who also apparently also suffered from mental illness had told the Mother to drug the children when they whined and cried. As if this was not enough, he was also found to be a criminal and was ordered out of the house in 2005 by the DSS for neglect, physical and sexual abuse but never left (Gray, 2007). A horrific and prime example of the infection of mental illness of the masses, were they themselves perhaps too hardened and/or too drugged themselves to see what was happening to the children and intervene to stop it? This is indeed an emotional epidemic, a sedation infection, a criminal complacency where one person after another in a chain of events looses the ability to know, realize, or see right from wrong.

The Whole Picture

When one looks at medications impact of the human body, one must also remember the medication that we do not choose or want to take, but do nonetheless. What I am talking about is "Pharmawater" the very real problem of 271 million pounds of pharmaceutical drugs in our water system. The Associated Press article called "Tons of released drugs taint US water" describes the serious problem of drug run off in our water system and how it is slowly destroying our eco-system, affecting both animals and humans alike.

This is no shocking news to me as I have long heard that birth control pills excreted in women's urine are flushed back into the water system and cause sterility among females and problems with males who chronically ingest sex-hormones through the tap. Add birth control pills with SSRIs, fluoride/aluminum, chlorine, 10,000 lbs of anti-biotics, explosive nitroglycerin, anti-convulsive phenytoin, left over chemo therapy drugs, and the anti-septic phenol-and you have a lethal drug cocktail that would make every human and animal a potential victim of a mass slow genocide. But have no fear, the drug companies assure us we are in no danger.

The drug companies that lobby for millions of dollars and drive around in $100,000 cars to offer goodies and vacations to American doctors, apparently have a "don't ask don't tell" policy on dumping their drugs. This is classic really, one of the scientists for the drug companies that was interviewed name was "Goldhammer" I thought that name was picturesque of what these big pharmaceutical companies are actually doing to the American people. Well here is Goldhammer's quote...do we laugh or cry?

"Goldhammer conceded some drug residues could be released in waste water, but stressed "it would not cause any environmental issues because it was not a toxic substance at the level that it was being released at"(Pritchard, 2009). While I appreciate Goldhammer's friendly spin on things and even the friendly name the epidemic is given which is "Pharmawater." But I choose to rename it the *Anna Nicole Syndrome*, the model/actress that died of a drug cocktail overdose, allegedly, steadily and sneakily mixed into her system by her friend/lawyer/lover and doctor- these people have now been indicted. Well, who will is going to indict the big pharmaceutical companies?

Of course, I hope for American's to heal themselves and release themselves from the death grip of the mighty monster pharmaceutical drug makers who suck their money, hide the cures, and keep them sick and begging for more but until that time comes I can hope for small changes everyday. A small few will rise up to take their lives and health back from this elite group who requires thrice day worship and a tithe of more than a quarter of the average American income!! There are 271 million pounds of different chemical drugs that you are swimming in, drinking, bathing in, eating, and drinking, if you think you have said "no" to drugs than think again. This means for every person on SSRIs already they could also theoretically be on several other drugs, unconsciously that interacts posing serious and deadly consequences.

Drugs, chemicals, and toxins all have a part to play in mental illness, although understand that I am saying too that mental illness has a psychological and genetic core and physical symptoms. This may sound like a strong statement but realize for me, as a doctor of natural health who believes in healing, it has to be so. If healing the core is an ultimate goal one cannot accept that circumstances are completely out of their own hands and that there is no hope. One has to believe in the power of change.

Healing the Mental Illness of Complacency

After my friend Francie died, I had wondered why I never contacted her and confronted her about some of the things she was writing, having seen some signs. For quite sometime I believed there was something wrong but I felt that I did not know her well enough to "stick my nose" into it. I now realize I had nothing to lose and I should have reached out in some way, rather than not at all. It also brings back to a story of a loved one. Someone close to me was on SSRIs and was stuck in a loathsome marriage and it got so bad that she didn't have food or heat for her child. She also lost her ability to work. I finally confronted her to get off of the drugs and take control of her life and when she did, all hell broke loose. A divorce ensued and a terrible custody battle. In this instance I realized that you can't just pull the plug on a drug, that there has to be a power within, a support system initiated, and a willingness to uncover what the drugs were covering up.

It is hard for me to admit, but I too had become complacent, many of us have become complacent. The causes are still something of a mystery; is it because of the violence on TV, pharmawater, fluoride water, childhood abuse, etc? At this point we can agree that it is what it is. A natural course of action for those combating mental instability in their life and others is to first combat the illness of complacency.

Healing Bi-Polar Disorder

The sky rocketing amount of people who have "bipolar" disorder in the states shows that this is a societal issue, just like autism, ADD and ADHD. More children are getting diagnosed, younger and younger as was the case with Rebecca Riley. What is "bi-polar?" This is an umbrella term and could very well be misinterpreted and misdiagnosed more often than not. However, term is a close relative to the very upsetting word "schizophrenia". The word "bi-polar" sounds friendlier and nicer but the word itself indicates a split in the personality and that is the very essence of schizophrenia.

The Orgonomist doctor that I interviewed told me that as much as 99.9% of the American population suffers from some degree of schizophrenia (Applebaum, 2003). The founder of Orgonomy, Wilhelm Reich, said that the most severe forms of schizophrenia manifest in the first seven days of life (Baker,1967). It has deep connections with how long a baby was kept from its mother following birth, birth trauma, such as circumcision and the stinging eye drops used at the moment of birth (which they don't use any more).

The slight degree of schizophrenia might be as simple as a case of chronic and habitual lying. This is actually incredibly common. For instance, consider the high school female who develops different personalities to meet parental and societal expectations. She might manage, somewhat successfully; one personality with the peers, one at school, another at church, and still another at home. Still this is on a somewhat conscious level, she knows she is doing and feels that she has to in order to survive. It could be as severe as violent attacks of mania and restrictive attacks of depression.

Bi-polar personality issues manifest as two polar opposites in the personality. The person literally fights "themselves" and fights to keep their true personality and emotions at bay. Part of the reason for this is because of parental and societal expectations, subjugation and sublimation tactics. Deeper emotional imbalances can only be helped by seeing a qualified Orgonomist doctor. The earlier schizophrenia is formed and the degree of the disorder, such as the case of a catatonic, the lesser the possibility of being completely healed (of course, anything is possible).

Clearing the mind and becoming more balanced and open to see more comprehensively and not selectively is an important first step for weeding out mental illness and keeping it in check. The course of ten years of studying, researching and testing out my own communication inadequacies has led me down a new path. I have devised in the following paragraphs as a grassroots approach to saving loved ones or even ourselves when we start to fall into mental instability.

In the Beginning

The beginning stages of mental illness can be hard to detect. One starts to "lose it" psychologically and then to their detriment, all of the people they love and trust fail to see it coming. People may start lying to and for them, even stroking their ego, and the person's sad process of falling into mental illness in the form of paranoia or delusional psychosis gets worse and worse until that person ultimately loses grip on reality. The next thing you know, the person you loved or befriended that acted a little off is psychologically and emotionally "gone."

I am not talking about severe psychosis here, but rather the workable degree of post modern neurosis of varying degrees termed "bi-polar" and formerly called "manic depression." Of course, severe mental illness is a process that takes years and years to completely take over. Instead of being detected and dealt with early on it can often be cemented by the person's immediate surroundings; family and friends. I call this the mental illness "Hiders," the people who pretend there is no problem to with the mentally and emotionally distraught person. This maybe also thought of as the easy way out, the hider does not have to emotionally enter and the ill person also becomes a hider and may in fact be consciously ok with the disconnective treatment. However, ignoring a problem doesn't mean the problem isn't there and will eventually go away. This is in some ways likened to the way people initially deal with an addictive person.

The Flip Side

There is such a phenomenon as the mental illness "holder." This unfortunate person is a family scapegoat and gets pinpointed as the "crazy" one. This Holder might in fact be *more* normal, *more* healthy and natural then the rest of the family but gets unduly elected as the "sick one." Sadly, this is just as common occurrence as the mental illness hiding. When advanced far enough it can actually lead to insanity if it was not already present and criminal behavior such as the ever so popular "teen angst" where children vandalize and destroy things.

    The biggest problem with these scenarios is that the core is ignored, relationship is sacrificed and all of the blame gets put on one person in the family structure. This disconnected approach proves minutely successful in group situations and holidays where you can hear the familial parent consoling themselves publicly, "I don't know what is wrong with -----, I did all I could for them." This again makes healing practically impossible because you have *the masses* posed as the family unit contributing to hysterical and divisive measures to keep control of the holder and yet remain in "good" standing within the community. Usually the holding takes place when a child's actions fall out of line of the parental standard and others around. When people such as family, neighbors, and church members start to become aware of the situation instead of the parent expanding and rallying behind their child; the parent instead views the child as embarrassing and so this method becomes employed sometimes radically as in institutionalizing or forced drugging to save face with the "world." Hence, it is not unusual for a "Hider" to quickly transform into a "Holder." More than that, it is plain to see that both situations were brought on by shame, embarrassment, and lying on the part of the parents.

The Role of Humanity

What causes us, as a race, to turn our backs on the people who should matter the most? It is that many of us are afraid to speak the truth or see the truth? We ignore the behavior or the bizarre symptoms or focus on one person and not the soul and core. In this way, mental illness diagnosis can become a crutch and a label that keeps people happily sedated and away from responsibility working in the benefit of the sick and the well. What are we *really* afraid of when dealing with the mentally ill?

Confrontation-Anger-Emotional Contact-and our own mental illness (Reich, 1972)

    I asked natural scientist and author of the book "Saharasia" Dr. James DeMeo what he thought about the use of pharmaceutical drugs in psychology and why humanity is following this path of drugs and mental illness here is what he said: "Dealing with human emotion, love and rage, not everyone can do it. Most ordinary people learn to bottle-up and live with it. Most professionals do also. They cannot go deeper; it is terrifying [to them]. It is therefore, so much easier to write prescriptions."

A True Friend is Truthful

I might offend people with this analogy, but I can think of no other better example than this. In the story of Christ we learn that he was a truthful, and thereby, a loyal friend. We know that part of his death and crucifixion was based on his truthfulness which was always based on intentions of love and healing. Yes, he cursed and swore at people and injustices; calling people vipers, liars, and hypocrites (Matt 23:13-39). He let people know the truth and steered away from complacency and yet he was fully and completely able to reach out and love them too (Matt 13:14, 15). In both instances he was showing the full range of human emotion. His hatred for the lie and his love of humanity were never once contracting or contradictory; in fact, he was always expanding in truth...even at the loss of his friends and life. This was made evident in the garden of Gethsemane when his closest friends would not stay awake for him. Then again when he was arrested and stood alone at the liberation of Barabas and his subsequent condemnation to death. Ironically a few days before, the same crowd that wanted to crown him king then turned their back and remained eerily silent in his defense (Matt 26 and 27).

So, You Realize Your Loved One is or Could be Mentally Ill.....

When you realize your spouse, parent, sibling or child is mentally ill it can bring up many different conflicting emotions within. Like the story of the emperor's new clothes, everyone else can see it or has had a glimpse of it at one time or another but pretends that they don't. Therefore, process becomes a game of hiding, lying, and pretending to protect the mentally ill person. You can--at any time--step out of the game. Realize that this is someone's life and they deserve a right to be healed.

Parental Roles in Mental Illness

Many parents of mentally ill children will go to great lengths to protect or hide the adult child's mental illness. What is the reason for this phenomenon? An overwhelming fear of being exposed *themselves*. A sick child is an open family wound and is strong evidence of parent's *perceived* inadequacies. This action by the parent to cover their tracks, so to speak, is sometimes called "love" but is inevitably fueled by emotions of guilt and shame. Any parent would understandably protest or become defensive thus making any progress in this area virtually impossible. This guilt/love for the child whether right or wrong does nothing to heal the child and may even help "spread the disease." The ability of a parent to both be strong, honest, and balanced is an absolute necessity if wellness is a goal.

The way parents handle adult mentally ill children stands in stark contrast to the way parents are now handling mentally ill children. There seems to be a bragging quality to it, even a bit of pride, that *they* think their child is mentally ill and so does *their* doctor so "bug off." I cannot tell you how much this disappoints me for reasons mentioned before as in Rebecca Riley's unfortunate situation. Time and time again I hear mothers explain to me that their child is bi-polar because their dad was, their uncle was, etc. More often than not this is pinned on the male children of the family. This leads me to believe that there very well could be a fear of the male or distrust of the male on part of the mother. They don't have to look at this possibility because they've got their prescriptions, they've a pat on the back from a family doctor and they have an audience which is the rest of the family that have become complacent. This is no small feat to overcome, but necessary nonetheless.

What is Friendship to You?

I ask you, is lying and deceiving people you care about being a friend? If you are a Christian, Muslim, Buddhist or Jew, is that course of action worthy of your religion? Are we going to keep following the path of Jesus's friends who lied and deserted him or are we going to seek the path of being honest and forthright thereby making a change for the future? Jesus started this trend over 2000 years ago and yet the world has yet come to embrace this. Forgive me, yes, Ghandi emulated Christ's example and it was through his communication with Leo Tolstoy on this subject which led to the freedom of the Indian people. But what about the rest of us, what about now?

Something Isn't Right, I Think…?

Don't doubt yourself or feel like you are talking about someone or judging when you start to realize a person is not "quite right."

It is up to you to: Live in truth, set an example, and be an honest friend

- Reach out and/or step away, depending on the situation: (You can present them with the truth, perhaps a suggestion and a solution but recognize that the person needs to accept and take control of their own life and they may need some alone time or to "contract" to process the information in order to hopefully "expand" at some point. Re-evaluate your motives for sticking so close in an unhealthy way, are you co-dependent? Are you a part of their sickness too? Don't be afraid to seek your own truth in a situation.

- Pray for and encourage your loved ones, whether silently from afar or as we sit near them. Sometimes this is all we can do and maybe a better alternative than sticking close to the person and habitually lying.

- Offer courses of action-don't just state the problem, be prepared to offer a solution. I always offer Orgonomy as I know this is a proven method to heal mental illness. Note: When offering to "drug" the person as a solution think whether or not the "band-aid" of pharmaceuticals will effectively remove the core of mental illness-it should be noted that the majority of antidepressants drugs contain heavy metals as inactive ingredients and fluoride/aluminum as an active ingredient which not only stores in the brain but renders its host emotionally numb and further from emotional contact. However, there is a point where drugging is necessary and the only course of action.

The fact is we are all suffering; this is the plight of humanity. We also know someone close to us that is emotionally suffering, no one escapes this truth which both unites us and separates us. We are also all to some degree mentally and emotionally "crippled" as a result of growing up in a nation where parents instead of setting examples and reaching out to their offspring left our emotional welfare to media and "others." With that being said, we can also check ourselves continually, making sure we are walking in truth and not disillusionment.

Our own human downfalls do need not be a hindrance to communication but a springboard. By connecting with others through our own truth, pain and imperfections, people are finally becoming more ready to listen and accept what is being shared. Being a friend to others is also speaking the truth in love. Our parents may not have been the finest examples for friendship and honesty but we can start now.

In this inspirational quote, Jesus quotes Isaiah:

"You shall indeed hear but never understand and you shall indeed see but never perceive. For this people's heart has grown dull [even duller with drug use], and their ears are heavy of hearing and their eyes they have closed, lest they should perceive with their hearts....and be healed" (Matt.13:14,15)

This is not a testament to religion I'm presenting here, but a true revelation that the same plague that rejected healing, love and acceptance 2,000 years ago is still infecting us today.

Naturopathic Psychotherapy, What is it?

Reich was the first scientist and psychologist to see the mind and body as one and to scientifically prove his findings. Furthermore, his work is the only psychotherapeutic model that is in keeping with the foundations of naturopathy. This means that only Orgonomy follows Dr. Henry Lindlahr's natural therapeutic laws of healing. Both Orgonomy and natural therapeutics [as stated and proved by Lindlahr] rely on expression and release for healing chronic emotional and physical disease.

In regards to expressing rather than suppressing Reich said, "In orgone therapy the [emotional/physical block] is loosened by means of biophysical methods and *not by means of psychological*. For the first time in the history of medicine...which is built and maintained by the fear of organ sensations, has found its medical opponent. This is our great obligation: TO ENABLE THE HUMAN ANIMAL TO ACCEPT NATURE WITHIN HIMSELF ...TO STOP RUNNING AWAY FROM IT. If we do not muster enough courage to maintain this insight we will fail as psychiatrists, physicians and educators." (Reich, 1972).

Conclusion

While I do not pretend to have all the answers to every illness, be it emotional or physical, I do believe emotional repression is a strong causal factor in all disease. To what extent? Everyone is different, but you can bet that careful self-examination and working through guiltless aggression would benefit everyone. We need to move past fear and move closer to health. Let us all take off the glasses of self illusion and begin to start looking at life and health more honestly. This involves a simple philosophical way to view our life. Are we actively engaged in life, or are we disengaged and out of touch with life? The goal must always be to come closer and make contact with ourselves and then with others.

Our western culture is on a pivotal brink of wellness and change. When we understand our selves, self-healing will become a dream finally realized and it will free us from the grips of the drug/vitamin companies. I also believe a talk with an honest friend can be a priceless healing treatment in and of it self. Any changes I have had in my own life came only when a dear friend challenged me and confronted me about a blindness I had in an area of my life. When that type of honest treatment comes to you, will you accept it or discard it because it came without a price tag? Will you listen and appreciate truth from someone who "knows too much" about you and has just as many issues as you? We must be willing to let down our defenses to love and heal, see and hear.

Remember the enchanting story of the "Little Prince"? In this story, due to a series of strange, magical events, the Little Prince finally learns about friendship and relationship by taming a fox. After he tames him, the fox gives him this secret: "One sees clearly only with the heart. Anything essential is invisible to the eyes."

May our hearts be healed and only then will our eyes be opened.

References

Ausubel, Kenny. (2000). *When healing becomes a crime.*
  Rochester: Healing Arts Press.

Ellerbe, Helen. (1995). *The dark side of Christian history.*
  Orlando: Morning Star & Lark.

Hamer, R. G. (2008). Excerpts from the summary of new medicine.
  Retrieved June 29, 2009, from http://www.newmedicine.ca
  Web site: http://www.newmedicine.ca/excerpt.php

Hunt, Valerie (2009). Emotional energy blocks to health and healing.
  Retrieved June 29, 2009, from http://www.bioenergyfields.org Web site:
  http://www.bioenergyfields.org/index.asp?secid=4&subsecid=0.

Herskowitz, Morton. (2001). *An introduction to psychiatric orgone therapy.*
  Piscataway: Transaction Publishers.

Demeo, James, Dr. (1998). *Saharasia.*
  Ashland: Natural Energy Works.

Miller, Neil. (1999). *Vaccines: are they really safe and effective?*
  Santa Fe: New Atantean Press.

Welch, Martha G. Dr. (1988). *Holding time.*
  New York: Simon and Schuster.

Reich, Wilhelm. (1983). *Children of the future.*
  Toronto: McGraw-Hill Ryerson, Ltd.

Liedloff, J. (1994). Who's in control. Retrieved June 29, 2009, from
  http://www.continuum-concept.org/ Web site:
  http://www.continuum-concept.org/reading/whosInControl.html

Acocella, J. (2000). The empty couch. *The New Yorker*, 112-118.

Doida, Brayman, Miller, Y, AA, MW. (1992). Modest enhancement of
  ultrasound- induced mutations in V79 cells in vitro.. Retrieved June 29,
  2009, from National Center for Biotechnology Information

Web site: http://www.ncbi.nlm.nih.gov/pubmed/
1509621?ordinalpos=1&itool=EntrezSystem2.PEntrez.Pubmed.
Pubmed_ResultsPanel.Pubmed_DiscoveryPanel.Pubmed_Discovery_
RA&linkpos=2&log$=relatedarticles&logdbfrom=pubmed

Rogers, C. (2006). Questions about prenatal ultrasound and the alarming increase in autism. Retrieved June 29, 2009, from http://www.midwiferytoday.com Website: http://www.midwiferytoday.com/articles/ultrasoundrodgers.asp

Wagner, M. (1999). Ultrasound: more harm than good?. Retrieved June 29, 2009, from http://www.midwiferytoday.com Web site: http://www.midwiferytoday.com/articles/ultrasoundwagner.asp

Wu, J. (2002). Sonic womb. Retrieved June 29, 2009, from http://www2.whdh.com Web site: http://www2.whdh.com/features/articles/healthcast/1893

Fatemi, M. (2006). The medical edge from the mayo clinic. Retrieved June 29, 2009, from http://www.mayo.edu Web site: http://www.mayo.edu/edge/c37.html.

Scott, J. (2009). Pesticides indicted in bee deaths. Retrieved June 29, 2009, from http://www.organicconsumers.org Web site: http://www.organicconsumers.org/articles/article_18017.cfm

Lindlahr, Henry. (1985). *Philosophy of Natural Therapeutics.* London: Vermilion.

Janakananda, Swami. (1992). *Yoga, tantra and meditation in daily life.* York Beach: Samuel Weiser, Inc.

Dinshah, Darius. (2005). *Let there be light.* Malaga: Dinshah Health Society.

Thirta, Shiva Swami Sada. (1998). *Ayurveda encyclopedia.* Bayville: Ayurveda Holistic Center Press.

Brennan, R. (2007). Fluorescent light ain't right. Retrieved June 30, 2009, from http://nymegaphone.com/ Web site: http://nyc.indymedia.org/en/2007/01/81805.html

References

Cousens, Gabriel, (2000). *Conscious eating.* Berkley: North Atlantic Books.

Farah, J. (2007, April 16). Consumers in dark over risks of new bulbs. Retrieved June 30, 2009, from www.worldnetdaily.com Web site: http://www.wnd.com/news/article.asp?ARTICLE_ID=55213

Sharma, Hari, M.D., Mishra Rama, G.A.M.S., Meade, & James G., Ph.D. (2002). *The answer to cancer.* New York: Select Books, Inc.

Hay, Louise L..(1999). *You can heal your life.* Carlsbad: Hay House, Inc.

Myss, Caroline, Ph.D..(2001*) Why people don't heal.* Colorado: Sounds True.

Upledger, John, D.O. (2002). *SomatoEmotional release.* Berkeley: North Atlantic Books.

Levey, Joel and Michelle. (1998). *Living in balance.* Berkeley: Conari Press.

Applebaum, Edward, D.O. (2004). *Conversation while driving from airport.* Farmington, MI.

Burrows, Stanley. (1993). *Healing for the age of enlightenment.* Auburn: Burroughs Books.

Gurudas. (1985). *Gem elixirs and vibrational healing, Vol. I.* San Rafael: Cassandra Press.

Golin, J. (2008, August 21). CCFC praises france baby TV ban; urges FTC action in the US. Retrieved June 30, 2009, from www.commercialexploitation.org Web site: http://www.commercialexploitation.org/pressreleases/babytvban.htm

Beaulieu, John, ND. (1995). *Music and sound in the healing arts.* New York: Station Hill Press.

Jordain, Robert. (2002). *Music, the brain and ecstasy.* New York: Harper Collins, Quills division.

Hitti, M. (2004, Oct. 13). Being bilingual boosts brain power. Retrieved
    June 30, 2009, from www.webmd.com
    Web site: http://www.webmd.com/parenting/news/20041013/
    being-bilingual-boosts-brain- power.

Diblassio, Brian (2008). Music Interview.
    Ann Arbor: Studio, questions in email.

Reich, Wilhelm, (1972). *Character analysis.*
    New York: Noonday Press.

Steenhuysen, J. (2009, May 5). More americans taking drugs for mental
    illness. Retrieved June 30, 2009, from http://www.reuters. com
    Web site: http://www.reuters.com/article/healthNews/
    idUSTRE5440V120090505

Cohen, E. (2007, July 9). CDC: antidepressants most prescribed in the U.S..
    Retrieved June 30, 2009, from CNN.com Web site:
    http://www.cnn.com/2007/HEALTH/07/09/antidepressants/index.html

Gallucci-White, G. (2009, April 22). Details emerge in Middletown
    family murder-suicide.. Retrieved June 30, 2009, from Frederick News
    Post Web site: www.fredericknewspost.com/sections/news/display.
    htm?storyID=89289

Cramer, Mishra, and Raja, (2007, Feb. 07). Girl fed fatal overdoses court told.
    Retrieved June 30, 2009, from Boston News
    Web site: http://www.boston.com/news/local/articles/2007/02/07/girl_
    fed_fatal_overdoses_court_told/

LaVoie, D. (2007, March 23). Mass. girl's overdose raises questions.
    Retrieved June 30, 2009, from USA Today Web site:
    http://www.usatoday.com/news/health/2007-03-23-drugged-to-
    death_N.htm

Gray, D. (2007, Feb. 23). The tragic death of rebecca riley.
    Retrieved June 30, 2009,from Health Central Web site:
    http://www.healthcentral.com/depression/c/18/6827/tragic-death-riley/

References

Pritchard, J. (2009, April 18). Tons of released drugs taint US water. Retrieved June 30, 2009, from News Yahoo Web site: http://news.yahoo.com/s/ap/20090419/ap_on_re_us/pharmawater_factories

Applebaum, Edward, D.O. (2004). *Conversation while driving from airport.* Farmington, MI.

Baker, Ellsworth. (1967). *Man in the trap.* New York: Macmillan Publishing co.

Reich, Wilhelm, (1972). *Character analysis.* New York: Noonday Press.

Demeo, James (2008). Email interview. March 20. Oregon: Naturalenergyworks.org

Bible, NKJV

Reich, Wilhelm, (1972). *Character analysis.* New York: Noonday Press.

De Saint Exupery, Antoine. (1943) *The little prince.* Florida: Harcourt, Inc.

Resources

Websites Orgonomy

http://www.orgonelab.org

Natural Homeschooling:

Kristie Karima Burns: Earthschooling/Waldorf inspired

http://waldorfenrichment.weebly.com/index.html

Rolfing (if you can't get to an Orgonomist or after Orgonomy)

Contact Jeff Belanger Annarborrolfing.com

Vaccines, Birth and Children's Health

http://909shot.com

http://www.midwiferytoday.com

http://www.birthworks.org

http://www.waldorfinthehome.com

http://mothering.com

http://www.vaclib.org/

Health

www.coopamerica.org (information on mad cow disease, poisonous cosmetics)

http://www.organicconsumers.org (become a member!)

http://www.vedicworld.org (Ayurveda and gem recommendations)

Books of Interest

Man in the Trap by Elsworth Baker M.D. The

Whole Mind by Lynette Bassman Ph.D The

Natural Pregnancy Book by Aviva Romm

The Magnetic Effect by Albert Roy Davis and Walter C. Rawls, Jr.

The Spirit of Homeopathic Medicines by Didier Grandgeorge

You are Your Child's First Teacher by Rahima Baldwin

Resources

A list of cosmetic companies that signed the "Compact for Safe Cosmetics" www.safecosmetics.org

* S, Akamuti — +0845-458-9242, www.akamuti.co.uk
* H S, Aubrey Organics — 800/237-4270, www.aubreyorganics.com/coop
* H S, Avalon Natural Products — www.avalonnaturalproducts.com
* H S M, Canary Cosmetics — www.canarycosmetics.com
* S, Dr. Bronner's Magic Soaps — 760/743-2211, www.drbronner.com
* S, Dropwise Essentials — 866/418-1682, www.dropwise.com
* S B, Earth Mama Angel Baby — 503/638-0487, www.earthmamaangelbaby.com
* H S M, EccoBella Botanicals — 877/696-2200, www.eccobella.com
* S, Eco-Beauty Organics — 208/267-9819, www.eco-beauty.com
* H, EcoColors — 877/852-4515, www.ecocolors.net
  * S M, Evan's Garden/Organic Beauty Inc. — 727/449-0900, www.evansgarden.com
* S, Farmaesthetics — 800/711-9194, www.farmaesthetics.com
* S, Ferlow Botannicals — 604/322-4080, www.ferlowbotanicals.com
* S M, Honeybee Gardens, Inc. — 610/396-9225, www.honeybeegardens.com
* H S, Inky Loves Nature — www.inkylovesnature.com
* S, Juice Beauty — 888/90-JUICE, www.juicebeauty.com
* S, Marie-Veronique Skin THerapy — www.m-vskintherapy.com
* H S, Max Green Alchemy Ltd. — 415/863-4155, www.maxgreenalchemy.com
* S, Moonshine Soap Co. — www.moonshinesoap.com
* S, Naturopathica Holistic Health — 800/592-7995 www.naturopathica.com
* S B, Plant Life, Inc. — 888/708-PURE, www.plantlife.net
* H S M B, Saffron Rouge, Inc. — 866/FACE-CARE, www.saffronrouge.com
* S, Sensua Organics — 800/983-1993, www.sensuaorganics.com

References

* S M, Sevi Cosmetics — 410/766-5151, www.sevikay.com
* H S, SMB Essentials/Lotus Moon Skin Care — 888/762-2667, www.lotusmoon.biz
* S, Spirit of Beauty — 425/453-0244, www.nutritionskincare.com
* H S, Spiritus Terrae — 877/PURITY2, www.naturepurity.com
* S, Sue's Slaves — www.suesalves.com
* S, Suki's Naturals — 888/858-SUKI, www.sukisnaturals.com
* M, Suncoat Products — 519/820-5468, www.suncoatproducts.com
* H S B, TerrEssentials — 301/371-7333,* S, Spirit of Beauty — 425/453-0244, www.nutritionskincare.com

Natural Products Companies That Are Also CABN Members

* S, A Wild Texas Soap Bar — 512/272-4058, www.awildtexassoapbar.com
* S, Indigo-Daisy-Shack — 702/807-6402, www.indigo-daisy-shack.com
* S, Osea Skin Care — 888/367-6732, www.oseaskin.com

Questions or Details on:

Herbs, Therapy and Detox?

Contact Aurore at:

Aurore@beyondnaturalmedicine.com

Visit her on the Web to find out about upcoming books and exciting new plans:

www.beyondnaturalmedicine.com

Ayurveda- Naturopathic Psychotherapy

**Color
and
Sound**

Made in the USA
Monee, IL
13 April 2021